Handwritten annotations:

TeCNU Extreme

VT vs SUt aberrancy

RBBB - $V_1 V_2$ - Brugada's Syndrome

will have Vtach arrest

$S_1 Q_3 T_3$ = PE

American Heart Association

Learn and Live SM

W9-BPM-457

Advanced Cardiovascular Life Support
PROVIDER·MANUAL

Editor

John M. Field, MD
Senior Science Editor

Associate Editors

Louis Gonzales, NREMT-P
Senior Oversight Editor
Mary Fran Hazinski, RN, MSN
Senior Science Editor

Special Contributors

Judy Ruple, PhD, RN, NREMT-P
Richard Talley, MD
Bob Elling, MPA, NREMT-P
Brenda Drummonds, ACLS Writer
Anthony Busti, PharmD
Michael Shuster, MD
Frank Doto, MS

ACLS Subcommittee 2005-2006

Terry L. Vanden Hoek, MD, Chair
Robert O'Connor, MD, Immediate Past
  Chair, 2004-2005
John E. Billi, MD
Henry R. Halperin, MD
Todd J. Crocco, MD
Steven Kronick, MD, MS
Mark S. Link, MD
Laurie Morrison, MD
Robert Neumar, MD
Mary Ann Peberdy, MD
Roger D. White, MD
Charles Otto, MD, PhD

Handwritten annotations:

intrinsic
primary - sinus 60-100
Escape AV junction 40-60
vent <40

Hypo vol
Hypoxia
H
↑↓ K^+
Hypothermia
Hypoglycemia

Toxicology
Ten PTX
Tamponade - Pericardial
Thrombosis - Coronary
Thrombosis - Pulm
Trauma

MAT 3 P waves of diff morphology
VT → 3 Beats

ISBN 0-87493-496-6
© 2006 American Heart Association

Best line → central

EPI 1 mg q 3 min
resus.

Vasopressin 400 IU

work above / below third

300 No pulse
150 c pulse

anti arrythm

Amiodarone — 300 IU VT/VF — K⁺/CA/BB-Blocker
IV push 1 mg/min drip
Lido 150 mg — max 300 mg 1/2/3 mg drip
works AV down — VT

Magnesium — 2 mg IV push

Procainamide — Na channel block 1–1.5 gm
30 mg/minute

Sodium Bicarb — acidosis
Not for code

Calcium — increases BP
Hypocalcemia
HyperKalemia (Calcium chloride)
more calcium

CPEA

Atropine — poisons vagus nerve
Dry secretions in mouth
1 mg × 3 — Max — then pace

Brady
Active Vagus Nerve
Damage AV/SA

MI
ACS
Drugs — BB/CCB/Digoxin

Brady
Atrope 1–23.
Parasym Nerve
Ø < 0.5
↑ HR Dopamine
10 mcg/kg
Kids → Epi 2–10 ug/min
trans cutaneous pace
Isoproterenol (Rare)
Beta-1-agonist.
Glucagon.
↓ antidote to BB or CCB overdose

ACLS Subcommittee 2004-2005

Robert O'Connor, MD, MPH, Chair
Max Harry Weil, MD, PhD, Immediate Past Chair, 2003-2004
Todd J.Crocco, MD
Terry L. Vanden Hoek, MD
John E. Billi, MD
Henry R. Halperin, MD
Edward C. Jauch, MD
Steven Kronick, MD, MS
Mary Ann Peberdy, MD
Charles Otto, MD, PhD
Dolores Kappel, RN
Rashmi Kothari, MD
Norman A. Paradis, MD
Edward M. Racht, MD

Acknowledgments

Peter Oluf Anderson, MD
Ulrik Christensen, MD

To find out about any updates or corrections to this text, visit www.americanheart.org/cpr and click on the "Course Materials" button.

ii

Contents

Student CD Contents

Note on Medication Doses

Emergency cardiovascular care is a dynamic science. Advances in treatment and drug therapies occur rapidly. Readers are advised to check for changes in recommended doses, indications, and contraindications in the following sources: *Currents in Emergency Cardiovascular Care,* which is available on the Worldwide Web at http://www.americanheart.org/cpr, the ECC Handbook, and the package insert product information sheet for each drug and medical device.

Considerations for International Readers

The following table is intended for international participants of this course. It is meant to help explain materials in this course that may be relevant only to those in the United States. For more specific information about your local practices and organizations please contact your instructor.

Page 34	In the *Airway Breathing Circulation* section, the compression depth is given in inches. Please note the following metric conversion: 1.5 to 2 inches = 4 to 5 centimeters
Page 37	In Step two of the section titled *The Universal AED: Common Steps to Operate All AEDs,* the placement of the pads is recommended to be "a few inches below the left armpit." Please refer to Figure 6 for a representation of this distance.
Page 104	In Figure 18, the Stroke Chain of Survival, the first link makes reference to the 911 emergency number. This system is specific to the US. Please contact your instructor regarding the emergency number system in your area.
Page 105	In the section titled *Foundation Facts,* the 911 telephone system is referenced. This system is specific to the US. Please contact your instructor regarding the emergency number system in your area.
Page 107	In the section titled *Activate EMS System Immediately,* the 911 telephone system is referenced. This system is specific to the US. Please contact your instructor regarding the emergency number system in your area.
Page 117	Under the heading titled *Pretreatment* in Table 8, the dosage for nitropaste is given in inches. Please note the following metric conversion: 1 to 2 inches = 2.5 to 5 centimeters

Part 1

Course Overview

Introduction

The Advanced Cardiovascular Life Support (ACLS) Provider Course is designed for health-care providers who either direct or participate in the resuscitation of a patient, whether in or out of hospital. In this course you will enhance your skills in the treatment of arrest and peri-arrest patients through active participation in a series of simulated cardiopulmonary cases. These simulations are designed to reinforce important concepts, including

- Identification and treatment of medical conditions that place the patient at risk for cardiac arrest
- The Basic Life Support (BLS) Primary Survey
- The ACLS Secondary Survey
- ACLS algorithms
- Effective resuscitation team dynamics

The goal of the ACLS Provider Course is to improve the quality of care provided to the adult victim of cardiac arrest or other cardiopulmonary emergencies.

Course Objectives

Upon successful completion of this course, you should be able to

- Recognize and initiate early management of peri-arrest conditions that may result in cardiac arrest or complicate resuscitation outcome
- Demonstrate proficiency in providing BLS care, including prioritizing chest compressions and integrating AED use
- Manage cardiac arrest until return of spontaneous circulation (ROSC), termination of resuscitation, or transfer of care
- Identify and treat ischemic chest pain and expedite the care of patients with acute coronary syndromes
- Recognize other life-threatening clinical situations, such as stroke, and provide effective initial care and transfer to reduce disability and death
- Demonstrate effective communication as a member or leader of a resuscitation team and recognize the impact of team dynamics on overall team performance

Course Description

To help you achieve these objectives, the ACLS Provider Course includes practice learning stations and a Megacode testing station.

The *practice learning stations* give you an opportunity to actively participate in a variety of learning activities, including

- Simulated clinical scenarios
- Demonstrations by instructors or video
- Discussion and role playing
- Practice in effective resuscitation team behaviors

In these learning stations you will practice essential skills both individually and as part of a team. This course emphasizes effective team skills as a vital part of the resuscitative effort. You will receive training in effective team behaviors and have the opportunity to practice as a team member and a team leader.

At the end of the course you will participate in a *Megacode testing station* to validate your achievement of the course objectives. A simulated cardiac arrest scenario will test the following:

- Knowledge of core case material and skills
- Knowledge of algorithms
- Understanding of arrhythmia interpretation
- Use of appropriate basic ACLS drug therapy
- Performance as an effective team leader

Course Materials

Course materials consist of the *ACLS Provider Manual* and the accompanying student CD. This icon directs you to additional supplemental information on the CD.

ACLS Provider Manual

The *ACLS Provider Manual* contains the basic information you need to know to effectively participate in the course. This important material includes the systematic approach to a cardiopulmonary emergency, effective resuscitation team communication, and the ACLS core cases and algorithms. *Please review this manual before attending the course. Bring it with you for use and reference during the course.*

The manual is organized into the following parts:

Part	Title	Content Summary
1	Course Overview	Course objectives, description, materials, prerequisites, preparation, and criteria for completion
2	BLS Primary Survey and ACLS Secondary Survey	Basic concepts and systematic approach to use in all cardiopulmonary emergencies
3	Effective Resuscitation Team Dynamics	Effective team behaviors to enhance resuscitation team performance
4	Core Cases	10 core patient care simulations

Student CD

The ACLS Provider Manual Supplementary CD (student CD) contains self-assessment and supplementary resources:

Resource	Description	How to use
ACLS Rhythm Identification	Self-assessment CD-based test: recognition of basic electrocardiogram (ECG) rhythms	Take *before the course* to help evaluate your proficiency and determine the need for remediation
ACLS Pharmacology	Self-assessment CD-based test: drugs used in algorithms	
Practical Application ACLS Algorithms	Self-assessment CD-based test: evaluates the practical application of rhythm recognition and pharmacology in the ACLS algorithms	
ACLS Supplementary Information	Supplementary resources: • Basic Airway Management • Advanced Airway Management • ACLS Core Rhythms • Defibrillation • Access for Medications • Acute Coronary Syndromes • Stroke • Medical Emergency Teams • Human, Ethical, and Legal Dimensions of ECC and ACLS	Additional information to supplement basic concepts presented in ACLS course. Some information is supplemental; other areas are for the interested learner or advanced provider
ACLS Core Drugs	Supplementary resources: information from the ECC Handbook on drugs used in the core cases	For review before taking the pharmacology self-assessment test; to remediate gaps in knowledge identified by self-assessment
BLS for Healthcare Providers Video Clips	Supplementary resources: selected video clips showing BLS skills.	To review BLS skills to prepare for the 1-rescuer CPR/AED testing station
ACLS Science Overview Video	Supplementary resources: video describing the core emphasis of the ACLS course from a science perspective	To update ACLS knowledge and learn about changes in application of ACLS science

Critical Concepts:

**Important
Information to
Review and Study**

Pay particular attention to the **Critical Concepts** boxes that appear in the *ACLS Provider Manual*. The concepts presented in these boxes are critical information that you need to know. You will also see **Foundation Facts** boxes. These boxes contain information that is basic to your understanding of the topics covered in the course. **FYI** boxes contain additional material "for your information."

Course Prerequisites and Preparation

The ACLS Provider Course is limited to healthcare providers who either will direct or participate in the resuscitation of a patient, either in or out of hospital. Participants who enter the course must have the basic knowledge and skills to actively participate with the instructor and other students in course activities.

Before the course, please read the ACLS Provider Manual, *complete the self-assessment modules (tests) on the student CD, identify any gaps in your knowledge, and remediate by studying applicable content in the* ACLS Provider Manual *or other supplementary resources.*

The following knowledge and skills are required for successful course completion:

- BLS skills
- ECG rhythm interpretation for core ACLS rhythms
- Basic ACLS drug and pharmacology knowledge
- Practical application of ACLS rhythms and drugs
- Effective resuscitation team concepts

BLS Skills

Strong BLS skills are the foundation of advanced life support. You must pass the 1-rescuer CPR/AED evaluation station to successfully complete the ACLS course. *Make sure that you are proficient in BLS skills before attending the course.*

Watch the video clips from the BLS for Healthcare Providers Course contained on the student CD. Review the CPR/AED Testing Checklist located in Appendix A.

ECG Rhythm Interpretation for Core ACLS Rhythms

You will need to know the monitor and paper tracing rhythms associated with basic cardiac arrest and peri-arrest algorithms. These rhythms are

- Sinus rhythm
- Atrial fibrillation and flutter
- Bradycardia
- Tachycardia
- Atrioventricular block
- Asystole
- Pulseless electrical activity (PEA)
- Ventricular tachycardia (VT)
- Ventricular fibrillation (VF)

Take the ECG rhythm identification self-assessment test on the student CD to evaluate your performance. At the end of the test you will receive your score and feedback to help you identify areas of strength and weakness. Remediate any gaps in your knowledge before entering the course. During the course you must be able to identify and interpret rhythms during practice as well as during the final Megacode testing station.

Basic ACLS Drug and Pharmacology Knowledge

You must know the pharmacology used in the ACLS algorithms. During the course you will be expected to know the drugs and doses used in the ACLS algorithms. You will also need to know *when* to use *which* drug based on the clinical situation.

Take the pharmacology ACLS review self-assessment test on the student CD to evaluate your performance. At the end of the test, you will receive your score and feedback to help you identify areas of strength and weakness. Remediate any gaps in your knowledge before entering the course. Resources for review of pharmacology are the ACLS Core Drug section on the student CD and the ACLS algorithms in the *ACLS Provider Manual*.

Practical Application of ACLS Rhythms and Drugs

Take the ACLS practical application self-assessment test on the student CD to evaluate your ability to integrate both rhythm interpretation and the use of pharmacologic agents. This test presents a clinical scenario and an ECG rhythm. You will need to take an action, give a specific drug, or direct your team to intervene. Use this self-assessment to confirm that you have the knowledge you need to be an active participant in the course and pass the final Megacode test.

Effective Resuscitation Team Concepts

Throughout the course you will be evaluated on your effectiveness as a team leader and a team member. A clear understanding of these concepts is integral to successful performance in the learning activities. Review Part 3 in the *ACLS Provider Manual* before the course. In the Megacode you will be evaluated using your team leader skills. A major emphasis of assessment will be your ability to direct the integration of BLS and ACLS by your team members.

Requirements for Successful Course Completion

To successfully complete the ACLS Provider Course and obtain your card, you must do the following:

- Pass the 1-rescuer CPR/AED testing station
- Participate, practice, and complete all learning stations
- Pass the Megacode testing station
- Pass the closed-book written exam with a minimum score of 84%

Part 2

The Systematic Approach: The BLS Primary Survey and ACLS Secondary Survey

Introduction

The goal of resuscitation interventions for a patient in respiratory or cardiac arrest is to support and restore effective oxygenation, ventilation, and circulation with return of intact neurologic function. An intermediate goal of resuscitation is the return of spontaneous circulation (ROSC). The actions used are guided by the following systematic ABCD approaches:

- BLS Primary Survey
- ACLS Secondary Survey

Learning Objectives

By the end of this part you should be able to

1. Describe the BLS Primary Survey and ACLS Secondary Survey with critical actions
2. Describe specific assessment and management that occur with each step of the systematic approach
3. Describe how you can apply this approach to almost all cardiopulmonary emergencies

The BLS Primary Survey

Overview of the BLS Primary Survey

The BLS Primary Survey is a systematic approach to basic life support. It can be performed by any trained healthcare provider. This approach stresses *early CPR* and *early defibrillation*. It does not include advanced interventions, such as advanced airway techniques or administration of drugs. The BLS goal is to support or restore effective oxygenation, ventilation, and circulation until ROSC or until ACLS interventions can be initiated. Performance of the actions in the BLS Primary Survey substantially improves a patient's chance of survival and a good (or better) neurologic outcome. **Before conducting the BLS Primary Survey, you should check patient responsiveness, activate EMS, and get an AED.**

The BLS Primary Survey is an ABCD approach using a series of sequential assessments. Each assessment is followed by appropriate action(s) if needed. As you *assess* each step (the patient's airway, breathing, circulation, and determine if defibrillation is needed), you stop and *perform an action*, if necessary, before proceeding to the next assessment step. Assessment is a key component in this approach. For example:

- Check breathing before giving rescue breaths or starting bag-mask ventilation, then
- Check the pulse before starting chest compressions or attaching an AED, then
- Analyze for a shockable rhythm before delivering a shock

> *Remember: assess...then perform appropriate action.*

Although the BLS Primary Survey requires no advanced equipment, use universal precautions and adjuncts that are readily available, such as a bag-mask ventilation device. The table below is an overview of the BLS Primary Survey. For more detail, review the *BLS for Healthcare Provider Student Manual* and watch the BLS Video Clips on the Student CD.

TABLE 1. The BLS Primary Survey

Assess	Action
Airway *–Is the airway open?*	Open the airway using noninvasive techniques (head tilt–chin lift or jaw thrust without head extension if trauma is suspected).
Breathing *–Is the patient breathing and are respirations adequate?*	Look, listen, and feel for adequate breathing. Give 2 rescue breaths. Give each breath over 1 second. Each breath should make the chest rise. Do not ventilate too fast (rate) or too much (volume).
Circulation *–Is a pulse present?*	Check carotid pulse for at least 5 seconds but no longer than 10 seconds. Perform high-quality CPR until an AED arrives.
Defibrillation *–If no pulse, check for a shockable rhythm with a manual defibrillator or use an AED.*	• Provide shocks as indicated. • Follow each shock immediately with CPR, beginning with chest compressions.

Critical Concepts:

Minimizing Interruptions

ACLS providers must make every effort to minimize any interruptions in chest compressions. Try to limit interruptions in chest compressions to no longer than 10 seconds except for specific interventions (eg, defibrillation, advanced airway or moving the patient from a dangerous environment). When you stop chest compressions, blood flow to the brain and heart decreases rapidly and stops.

Avoid:

- Prolonged rhythm analysis
- Frequent or inappropriate pulse checks
- Taking too long to give breaths to the patient
- Unnecessarily moving the patient

The ACLS Secondary Survey

Overview of Secondary Survey

The ACLS Secondary Survey is conducted after the BLS Primary Survey when more advanced, invasive assessment and management techniques are needed. Advanced airway interventions may include the Combitube, laryngeal mask airway (LMA), or endotracheal intubation. Advanced circulatory interventions may include drugs to control heart rhythm and blood pressure. An important component of this survey is the differential diagnosis, where identification and treatment of the underlying causes may be critical to patient outcome.

In the ACLS Secondary Survey, you continue to assess and perform an action as appropriate until transfer to the next level of care. Many times assessments and actions in ACLS will be performed simultaneously by team members.

Remember: assess ...then perform appropriate action.

The table below is an overview of the ACLS Secondary Survey. The components are discussed in greater detail in Part 4: ACLS Core Cases.

TABLE 2. The ACLS Secondary Survey

Assess	Action as Appropriate
Airway –*Is the airway patent?* –*Is an advanced airway indicated?*	• Maintain airway patency in unconscious patients by use of head tilt–chin lift, oropharyngeal airway (OPA), or nasopharyngeal airway (NPA). • Use advanced airway management if needed (eg, LMA, Combitube, endotracheal intubation).

Breathing
 	
–*Are oxygenation and ventilation adequate?*
 	
–*Is an advanced airway indicated?*
 	
–*Is proper placement of airway device confirmed?*
 	
–*Is tube secured and placement reconfirmed frequently?*
 	
–*Are exhaled CO_2 and oxyhemoglobin saturation monitored?*
	• Give supplementary oxygen.
	• Assess the adequacy of oxygenation and ventilation by
	  — Clinical criteria (chest rise)
	  — Oxygen saturation
	  — Capnometry or capnography
	
	The benefit of advanced airway placement is weighed against the adverse effect of interrupting chest compressions. If bag-mask ventilation is adequate, insertion of an advanced airway may be deferred until the patient fails to respond to initial CPR and defibrillation or until spontaneous circulation returns.
	
	If advanced airway devices are used:
	
	• Confirm proper integration of CPR and ventilation.
	• Confirm proper placement of advanced airway devices by
	  — Physical examination
	  — Measurement of exhaled CO_2
	  — Use of esophageal detector device
	• Secure the device to prevent dislodgment.
	• Continue exhaled CO_2 measurement.

Circulation –*What was the initial cardiac rhythm?* –*What is the current cardiac rhythm?* –*Have you established access for drug and fluid administration?* –*Does the patient need volume (fluid) for resuscitation?* –*Are medications needed for rhythm or blood pressure?*	• Obtain IV/IO access. • Attach ECG leads and monitor for arrhythmias or cardiac arrest rhythms (eg, VF, pulseless VT, asystole, and PEA). • Give appropriate drugs to manage rhythm (eg, amiodarone, lidocaine, atropine, magnesium) and blood pressure (eg, epinephrine, vasopressin, and dopamine). • Give IV/IO fluids if needed.

Assess	Action as Appropriate
Differential **D**iagnosis –*Why did this patient develop cardiac arrest?* –*Why is the patient still in arrest?* –*Can we identify a reversible cause of this arrest?*	• Search for, find, and treat reversible causes (ie, definitive care).

Part 3

Effective Resuscitation Team Dynamics

Introduction

Many tasks must be performed during resuscitation. A patient who has not been successfully resuscitated by a single CPR-trained bystander in the first moments after collapse can rarely be adequately managed by the addition of a single ACLS provider. This is where teamwork comes in. Teamwork divides the tasks while multiplying the chances of a successful resuscitation.

Successful teams not only have medical expertise and mastery of resuscitation skills, but they also demonstrate effective communication and team dynamics. Part 3 of this manual discusses the importance of team roles, behaviors of effective team leaders and team members, and elements of effective resuscitation team dynamics.

During the course you will have an opportunity to practice performing different roles as a member and leader of a simulated resuscitation team, including the role of a team leader.

Learning Objectives

By the end of this part, you should be able to

1. Explain the importance of team members understanding not only their roles but also the role of the team leader
2. Explain the importance of the team leader's understanding not only his or her role but also the role of team members
3. Explain why the foundation of successful resuscitations includes both mastery of basic skills *and* effective team dynamics
4. Describe the important elements of effective resuscitation team dynamics

Foundation Facts:

Understanding Team Roles

Whether you are a team member or team leader during a resuscitation attempt, you should *understand not only your role but also the roles of other members on your team.* This awareness will help you anticipate

- What actions will be performed next
- How to communicate and work as a member or leader of the team

Roles of the Team Leader and Team Members

Role of the Team Leader

The role of the team leader is multi-faceted. The team leader

- Organizes the group
- Monitors individual performance of team members
- Backs up team members
- Models excellent team behavior
- Trains and coaches
- Facilitates understanding
- Focuses on comprehensive patient care

Every resuscitation team needs a leader to organize the efforts of the group. The team leader is responsible for making sure everything gets done at the right time in the right way by monitoring and integrating individual performance of team members. The role of the team leader is similar to that of an orchestra conductor directing individual musicians. Like a conductor, the team leader does not play the instruments but instead knows how each member of the orchestra fits into the overall music.

However, the team leader must be proficient in all the specific skills that need to be accomplished during the resuscitation. This level of expertise is necessary because occasionally the team leader serves as a backup for a team member who may be having trouble performing her role or assigned task.

The role of the team leader also includes modeling excellent team behavior and leadership skills for the team and other people who may be involved or interested in the resuscitation. The team leader should serve as a teacher or guide to help train future team leaders and improve team effectiveness. After resuscitation the team leader can provide analysis, critique, and practice in preparation for the next resuscitation attempt.

The team leader also helps team members understand why certain tasks are performed in a specific way. The team leader should be able to explain to the team why it is essential to "minimize interruptions in chest compressions," "push hard and fast," "ensure full chest recoil," and "ventilate, not hyperventilate!" Review the ACLS Science Overview video on the Student CD to help prepare for this role.

Whereas team members focus on their individual tasks, the team leader is attentive to comprehensive patient care.

Role of the Team Member

Team members must be proficient in the skills they are trained and authorized to perform within their scope of practice. It is essential to the success of the resuscitation attempt that team members are

- Clear about role assignments
- Prepared to fulfill role responsibilities
- Well practiced in resuscitation skills
- Knowledgeable about the algorithms
- Committed to success

If it is not your responsibility to "run" the resuscitation as a team leader, then it is understandable that you may not have mastered all the specific tasks, such as selecting medications, interpreting rhythms, or making medical decisions. But it is expected that you will have mastered your areas of responsibility and will be committed to the success of the resuscitation attempt.

Elements of Effective Resuscitation Team Dynamics

1
Closed-Loop Communication

When communicating with resuscitation team members, the team leader should use closed-loop communication by taking these steps:

1. The team leader gives a message, order, or assignment to a team member.
2. The team leader confirms that the message was heard and understood by receiving a clear response and good eye contact from the team member.
3. The team leader listens for confirmation from the team member that the task was performed before assigning another task.

Do

Team Leader	Assign another task after receiving oral confirmation that a task has been completed, such as "Good, now that the IV is in, give 1 mg of epinephrine."
Team Members	Inform the team leader when a task begins or ends, such as "The IV is in."

Don't

Team Leader	Give more tasks without asking or receiving confirmation of a completed assignment
Team Members	• Give drugs without notifying or orally confirming the order with the team leader • Forget to report back that the drug has been given or the procedure has been performed • Start speaking without confirming that you clearly received the message

2
Clear Messages

Clear messages consist of concise communication spoken with distinctive speech in a controlled tone of voice. All messages and orders should be delivered in a calm and direct manner without yelling or shouting. Communication that is unclear can lead to unnecessary delays in treatment or to medication errors. For example: "Did the patient get IV propofol so I can proceed with the cardioversion?" "No, I thought you said to give him *propranolol*."

Yelling or shouting can impair effective team interaction. Only one person should be talking at any time.

Do

Team Leader	Encourage team members to speak clearly
Team Members	• Repeat the prescription medication order • Question an order if the slightest doubt exists

Don't

Team Leader	• Mumble or speak in incomplete sentences • Give unclear messages and prescription drug orders • Yell, scream, or shout
Team Members	Feel patronized by distinct and concise messages

3

Clear Roles and Responsibilities

Every member of the team should know his or her role and responsibilities. Just as different shaped pieces make up a jigsaw puzzle, each team member's role is unique and critical to the effective performance of the team. When roles are unclear, team performance suffers. Signs of unclear roles include

- Performing the same task more than once
- Missing essential tasks
- Freelancing of team members

To avoid inefficiencies the team leader should clearly delegate tasks. Team members should communicate when and if they can handle additional responsibilities. The team leader should encourage team members to participate in leadership and not simply follow directions blindly.

Do

Team Leader	Clearly define all roles of team members in the clinical setting
Team Members	• Seek out and perform tasks that are clearly defined and appropriate to your level of competence • Ask for a new task or role if your task is too difficult for you to perform based on your experience or competence

Don't

Team Leader	• Neglect to assign tasks to team members who are available • Assign tasks to team members who are unsure of their responsibilities • Distribute assignments unevenly leaving some with too much to do and others with too little
Team Members	• Avoid taking assignments • Take assignments beyond your level of competence or expertise

4

Knowing One's Limitations

Not only should everyone on the team know his or her own limitations and capabilities, but also the team leader should be aware of them. This knowledge allows the team leader to evaluate team resources and call for backup of team members when assistance is needed. Team members should anticipate situations in which they might require assistance and inform the team leader.

During the stress of an attempted resuscitation do not practice or explore a new skill. If extra help will be needed, request it early. Remember that it is not a sign of weakness or incompetence to call for help; it is better to have more help than needed rather than not enough help, which might negatively affect patient outcome.

Do

Team Leader and Team Members	• Call for assistance at an early stage rather than waiting until the patient deteriorates to the point that help is critical • Seek advice from more experienced personnel when the patient's condition worsens despite primary treatment

Don't

Team Leader and Team Members	Reject offers from others to carry out an assigned task you are unable to complete because of other activities —even though completion of the task is essential to treatment
Team Members	• Use or start an unfamiliar treatment or therapy without seeking advice from more experienced personnel • Take on too many assignments at a time when assistance is readily available

5

Knowledge Sharing

Sharing information is a critical component of effective team performance. Team leaders may become trapped in a specific treatment or diagnostic approach. Three common types of narrow-focus errors (also called fixation errors) are

- "Everything is okay"
- "This and only this is the correct path"
- "Anything but this"

When resuscitative efforts are ineffective, go back to the basics and talk as a team. "Well, we've gotten the following on the ACLS Secondary Survey…. Have we missed something?" Team members should inform the team leader of any changes in the patient's condition to ensure that decisions are made with all available information.

Do

Team Leader	• Encourage an environment of information sharing and ask for suggestions if uncertain of the next best interventions • Ask for good ideas for differential diagnoses • Ask if anything has been overlooked (eg, IV access should have been obtained or drugs should have been administered)
Team Member	Share information with other team members

Don't

Team Leader	• Ignore others' suggestions for treatment • Overlook or fail to examine clinical signs that are relevant to the treatment
Team Member	Ignore important information to improve your role

6

Constructive Intervention

During a resuscitation attempt, the team leader or a team member may need to intervene if an action that is about to occur may be inappropriate at the time. Constructive intervention is necessary but should be done tactfully. Team leaders should avoid confrontation with team members. Instead, conduct a debriefing afterwards if constructive criticism is needed.

Do

Team Leader	Ask that a different intervention be started if it has a higher priority
Team Members	• Suggest an alternative drug or dose in a confident manner • Question a colleague who is about to make a mistake

Don't

Team Leader	Fail to reassign a team member who is trying to function beyond his or her level of skill
Team Members	Ignore a team member who is about to administer a drug incorrectly

7

Reevaluation and Summarizing

An essential role of the team leader is monitoring and reevaluating

- The patient's status
- Interventions that have been performed
- Assessment findings

A good practice is for the team leader to summarize this information out loud in a periodic update to the team. Review the status of the resuscitation attempt and announce the plan for the next few steps. Remember that the patient's condition can change. Remain flexible to changing treatment plans and revisiting the initial differential diagnosis. Ask for information and summaries from the code recorder as well.

Do

Team Leader	• Draw continuous attention to decisions about differential diagnoses • Review or maintain an ongoing record of drugs and treatments administered and the patient's response
Team Leader and Team Members	Clearly draw attention to significant changes in the patient's clinical condition and increase monitoring (eg, frequency of respirations and blood pressure) when the patient's condition deteriorates

Don't

Team Leader	• Fail to change a treatment strategy although new information supports such a change • Fail to inform arriving personnel of the current status and plans for further action

8

Mutual Respect

The best teams are composed of members who share a mutual respect for each other and work together in a collegial, supportive manner. To have a high-performing resuscitation team everyone must leave his ego at the door and respect each other during the resuscitation attempt, regardless of any additional training or experience that the team leader or specific team members may have.

Do

Team Leader and Team Members	• Speak in a friendly, controlled tone of voice • Avoid shouting or displaying aggression if you are not understood initially
Team Leader	Acknowledge assignments that have been carried out correctly by saying "Thanks, good job!"

Don't

Team Leader and Team Members	• Shout or yell at team members—when one person raises his voice, others will do so too • Behave aggressively, by confusing directive behavior with aggression • Be uninterested in others

---

Foundation Facts:

Medical Emergency Teams (METs)

Rapid Response Teams (RRTs)

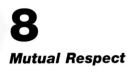

Medical emergency teams (METs) or Rapid Response Teams (RRTs) have been implemented in many hospitals. The purpose of these teams is to improve patient outcomes by identifying and treating early clinical deterioration. In-hospital cardiac arrest is commonly preceded by physiologic changes. In one study, nearly 80% of hospitalized patients with cardiorespiratory arrest had abnormal vital signs documented for up to 8 hours before the actual arrest. Many of these changes can be recognized by monitoring routine vital signs. Intervention before clinical deterioration or cardiac arrest may be possible.

Consider the question asked in the ACLS Experienced Provider Course: "Would you have done anything differently if you knew 15 minutes before the arrest that ...?"

Learn more about the evolving concept of medical emergency teams from the student CD.

Part 4

The ACLS Core Cases

Overview of the Core Cases

The ACLS core simulated cases are designed to review the knowledge and skills that you will need to successfully participate in course events and pass the Megacode. Each case contains the following topics:

- Introduction
- Learning objectives
- Rhythms and drugs
- Descriptions or definitions of key concepts
- Overview of algorithm
- Algorithm figure
- Application of the algorithm to the case
- Other related topics

This part contains the following cases.

Respiratory Arrest Case

Introduction	This case reviews appropriate assessment, intervention, and management options for an *unconscious, unresponsive adult patient in respiratory arrest. Respirations are completely absent or clearly inadequate to maintain effective oxygenation and ventilation. A pulse is present.* (Do not confuse agonal gasps with adequate respirations.) The BLS Primary Survey and the ACLS Secondary Survey are used even though the patient is in respiratory arrest and not in cardiac arrest.

Learning Objectives

At the end of this case, you will be able to

1. Describe use of the BLS Primary and ACLS Secondary Surveys in a patient in respiratory arrest with a pulse
2. Describe the clinical situations in which the following airway adjuncts may be used for airway management:

   - Oropharyngeal airway (OPA)
   - Nasopharyngeal airway (NPA)
   - Bag-mask ventilation
   - Advanced airway

Case Drugs

This case involves the following drugs:

- Oxygen

Additional drugs may be considered in systems or facilities where rapid-sequence intubation is performed. Refer to the ACLS Experienced Provider (EP) Course for a detailed discussion of this procedure.

The BLS Primary Survey

First Steps

The first steps in treating any emergency before assessing ABCDs are

Step	Action
Scene safety	Make sure the scene is safe for you and the victim. You do not want to become a victim yourself
Check response	Tap the victim's shoulder and shout, "Are you all right?"
Activate the emergency response system	• If you are alone, shout for help. • If no one responds, activate the emergency response system, phone 911 or emergency number, and • Get an AED if available. • Then return to the victim and begin CPR.

Foundation Fact: **Lone HCP May** **Tailor Response**	Lone healthcare providers may tailor the sequence of actions to the most likely cause of arrest. For patients with a likely asphyxial arrest, the lone rescuer should perform 2 minutes (about 5 cycles) of CPR before leaving the patient to activate the emergency response system and get an AED. Then return to the patient, resume CPR, and use the AED if indicated.

ABCD Assessment

Then proceed with the ABCD assessment of the BLS Primary Survey as described below.

Assess	Action
Airway	**Open the airway using noninvasive techniques:** • Head tilt–chin lift *or* • Jaw lift without head extension if trauma is present or suspected **While observing the patient's chest:** • ***Look*** for the chest to rise and fall. • ***Listen*** for air escaping during exhalation. • ***Feel*** for flow of air against your cheek.
Breathing	If respirations are absent or inadequate: **Give 2 breaths.** Use a barrier device if available. Each breath should take 1 second and cause visible chest rise.
Circulation	**Feel for a carotid pulse for at least 5 seconds but no more than 10 seconds.** Note: In this case the patient has a pulse, and chest compressions are not indicated.
Defibrillation	**If no pulse, attach an AED or manual defibrillator.** Follow AED prompts or shock if indicated. Note: In this case (respiratory arrest with a pulse) the AED is not attached.

Note that the BLS Primary Survey focuses on early CPR and early defibrillation. Intravenous/intraosseous (IV/IO) access is not discussed here even though medications may provide a clinical benefit to some patients. Advanced assessments and interventions are part of the ACLS Secondary Survey.

The patient in this case will not require chest compressions or defibrillation. Because this patient has a pulse, do not power on the AED or apply the defibrillator pads.

Assess and Reassess the Patient

The systematic approach of the BLS Primary Survey is *assessment* then *action* for each step of the ABCD sequence.

> *Remember: assess...then perform appropriate action.*

In this case you assess and find that the patient has a pulse, so you do not use the AED or begin chest compressions. During the course your instructor will emphasize the need to re-assess the patient and be ready to do CPR, attach the AED, and shock the patient if indicated.

Ventilation and Pulse Check

For a patient in respiratory arrest with a pulse, give 1 breath about every 5 to 6 seconds or 10 to 12 breaths per minute. Recheck the pulse about every 2 minutes. Take at least 5 seconds but no more than 10 seconds for a pulse check.

The ACLS Secondary Survey

Airway Management in Respiratory Arrest

In the management of respiratory arrest skills station, you will have an opportunity to practice critical skills for assessing and managing the airway. You will

- Demonstrate correct placement of an OPA and NPA
- Perform bag-mask ventilation
- Become familiar with advanced airway equipment
- Learn how to ventilate when an advanced airway is in place

FYI	The ACLS Provider Course will familiarize you with advanced airway equipment, but you will not learn or practice insertion. You will, however, practice and perform integration of ventilation and chest compressions with an endotracheal (ET) tube in place. Advanced airway equipment includes the esophageal-tracheal Combitube, the laryngeal mask airway (LMA), and the ET tube.

The decision to place an advanced airway is made during the ACLS Secondary Survey. If a patient is in cardiac arrest, placement of an advanced airway may interrupt chest compressions for many seconds. The need for compressions is weighed against the need for an advanced airway. If bag-mask ventilation is adequate, insertion of an advanced airway may be deferred until the patient fails to respond to initial CPR and defibrillation or until spontaneous circulation returns.

Below is a summary of the ACLS Secondary Survey applied to this case.

Assess	Determine Management as Appropriate
Airway	- Maintain airway patency in unconscious patients by use of head tilt–chin lift, oropharyngeal airway (OPA), or nasopharyngeal airway (NPA). - Use advanced airway management if needed (eg, LMA, Combitube, endotracheal intubation).
Breathing	- Give bag-mask ventilations every 5 to 6 seconds—about 10 to 12 breaths per minute (rescue breathing without chest compressions). The benefit of advanced airway placement is weighed against the adverse effect of interrupting chest compressions. If bag-mask ventilation is adequate, insertion of an advanced airway may be deferred until the patient fails to respond to initial CPR and defibrillation or until spontaneous circulation returns. If advanced airway devices are used: - **Confirm placement of advanced airway** device by a physical examination and a confirmation device (exhaled CO_2 detector, esophageal detector device). - **Secure the advanced airway device** to prevent dislodgment, especially in patients at risk for movement. Secure the ET tube with tape or a commercial device. Consider capnography; continuous quantitative end-tidal CO_2 monitor display.

Assess	Determine Management as Appropriate
Circulation	• **Obtain IV/IO access** • **Attach ECG leads** • **Identify and monitor for arrhythmias** (eg, VF, pulseless VT, asystole, PEA, symptomatic bradycardia, and tachycardia) • **Give fluids if indicated**
Differential **D**iagnosis	**Search for, find, and treat** reversible causes and contributing factors.

Ventilations

In this case the patient is in respiratory arrest, so ventilate the patient **once every 5 to 6 seconds** or 10 to 12 times per minute. Each breath should take 1 second and achieve visible chest rise. Be careful to avoid excessive ventilations (too many breaths per minute or too large a volume per breath).

Management of Respiratory Arrest

Overview

Management of respiratory arrest includes both BLS and ACLS interventions. These interventions may include

- Giving supplementary oxygen
- Opening the airway
- Providing basic ventilation
- Using basic airway adjuncts (OPA and NPA)
- Suctioning
- Providing ventilation with advanced airways

> According to the 2005 guidelines, for patients with a perfusing rhythm, deliver **1 breath every 5 to 6 seconds** (10 to 12 breaths per minute).

Take special precautions when providing ventilation for patients with suspected cervical spine trauma. These precautions are discussed at the end of this section.

Critical Concepts:

Avoiding Hyperventilation

Whenever any form of assisted ventilation is used, you must be careful to avoid delivering too much ventilation (too many breaths or too large a volume). Hyperventilation (too many breaths per minute or too large a volume per breath) can be harmful because it increases intrathoracic pressure, decreases venous return to the heart, and diminishes cardiac output. It may also increase gastric inflation and predispose the patient to vomiting and aspiration of gastric contents.

Giving Supplementary Oxygen

Maintain Oxygen Saturation

Give oxygen to patients with acute cardiac symptoms or respiratory distress. Monitor oxygen saturation and titrate supplementary oxygen to maintain a saturation of at least 90%. Administer oxygen continuously if saturation is less than 90%.

Use of Oxygen and Monitoring of Equipment and Oxygen Flow

See the student CD for details on use of oxygen in patients not in respiratory or cardiac arrest.

Opening the Airway

Common Cause of Airway Obstruction

The most common cause of upper airway obstruction in the unresponsive patient is loss of tone in the throat muscles. In this case the tongue falls back and occludes the airway at the level of the pharynx (Figure 1A).

Basic Airway Opening Techniques

Basic airway opening techniques will be effective if the airway obstruction is caused by either the tongue or from relaxation of muscles in the upper airway. The basic airway opening technique is head tilt with anterior displacement of the mandible, ie, head tilt–chin lift (Figure 1B).

In the trauma patient with suspected neck injury, use jaw thrust without head extension (Figure 1C). Because maintaining an open airway and providing ventilation is a priority, use a head tilt–chin lift maneuver if the jaw thrust does not open the airway. ACLS providers should be aware that lay providers are no longer taught the jaw thrust technique.

Airway Management

Proper airway positioning may be all that is required for patients who can breathe spontaneously. In patients who are unconscious with no cough or gag reflex, insert an OPA or NPA to maintain airway patency.

If you find an unresponsive patient who was known to be choking and is now unresponsive and in respiratory arrest, open the mouth wide and look for a foreign object. If you see one, remove it with your fingers. If you do not see a foreign object, begin CPR. Each time you open the airway to give breaths, open the mouth wide and look for a foreign object. Remove it with your fingers if present. If there is no foreign object, resume CPR.

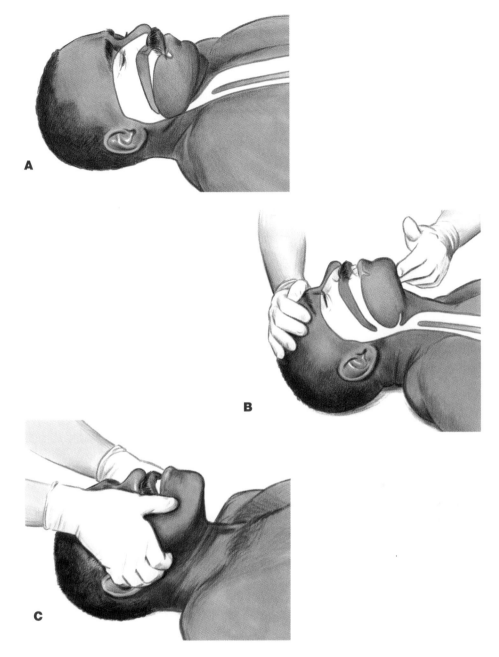

Figure 1. Obstruction of the airway by the tongue and epiglottis. When a patient is unresponsive, the tongue can obstruct the airway. The head tilt–chin lift relieves obstruction in the unresponsive patient. **A**, The tongue is obstructing the airway. **B**, The head tilt–chin lift maneuver lifts the tongue, relieving the obstruction. **C**, The jaw thrust without head extension is used if cervical spine trauma is suspected.

Providing Basic Ventilation

Basic Airway Skills

Basic airway skills used to ventilate a patient are

- Head tilt–chin lift
- Jaw thrust without head extension (suspected cervical spine trauma)
- Mouth-to-mouth ventilation
- Mouth-to-nose ventilation
- Mouth-to–barrier device (using a pocket mask)
- Bag-mask ventilation

For detailed information on these BLS skills, refer to the *BLS for Healthcare Providers Student Manual.*

Bag-Mask Ventilation

A bag-mask ventilation device consists of a ventilation bag attached to a face mask. These devices have been a mainstay of emergency ventilation for decades. Bag-mask devices are the most common method of providing positive-pressure ventilation.

The universal connections present on all interconnecting airway devices allow you to connect any ventilation bag to numerous adjuncts. Valves and ports may include

- 1-way valves to prevent the patient from rebreathing exhaled air
- Oxygen ports for administering supplementary oxygen
- Medication ports for administering aerosolized and other medications
- Suction ports for clearing the airway
- Ports for quantitative sampling of end-tidal CO_2

You can attach other adjuncts to the patient end of the valve, including a pocket face mask, ET tube, LMA, and Combitube.

See the Student CD for more information on bag-mask ventilation.

Basic Airway Adjuncts: Oropharyngeal Airway

Introduction

The oropharyngeal airway (OPA) is used in patients who are at risk for development of airway obstruction from the tongue or from relaxed upper airway muscles. This J-shaped device (Figure 2A) fits over the tongue to hold it and the soft hypopharyngeal structures away from the posterior wall of the pharynx.

The OPA is used in *unconscious* patients if procedures to open the airway (eg, head tilt–chin lift or jaw thrust) fail to provide and maintain a clear, unobstructed airway. An OPA *should not be used in a conscious or semiconscious patient* because it may stimulate gagging and vomiting. The key assessment is to check whether the patient has an intact cough and gag reflex. If so, do not use an OPA.

The OPA may be used to keep the airway open during bag-mask ventilation when rescuers might unknowingly push down on the chin, blocking the airway. The OPA is also used during suctioning of the mouth and throat and in intubated patients to prevent them from biting and occluding the ET tube.

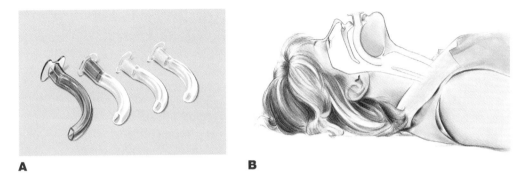

Figure 2. Oropharyngeal airways. **A,** Four oropharyngeal airway devices; **B,** One oropharyngeal airway device inserted.

Technique of OPA Insertion

Step	Action
1	**Clear the mouth and pharynx** of secretions, blood, or vomit using a rigid pharyngeal suction tip if possible.
2	**Select the proper size OPA.** Place the OPA against the side of the face. When the tip of the OPA is at the corner of the mouth, the phalange is at the angle of the mandible. When the OPA is properly sized and inserted, this results in proper alignment with the glottic opening.
3	**Insert the OPA** so that it is turned *backward* as it enters the mouth.
4	As the OPA passes through the oral cavity and approaches the posterior wall of the pharynx, **rotate it 180 degrees** into proper position (Figure 2B). An **alternative method** is to insert the OPA straight in while using a tongue depressor or similar device to hold the tongue on the floor of the mouth.

After insertion of an OPA, monitor the patient. Keep the head and jaw positioned properly to maintain a patent airway. Suction the airway as needed.

Cautions

Be aware of the following when using an OPA:

- If the OPA selected is *too* large, it may obstruct the larynx or cause trauma to the laryngeal structures.
- If the OPA is *too small* or is inserted improperly, it may push the base of the tongue posteriorly and obstruct the airway.
- Insert carefully to avoid soft tissue trauma to the lips and tongue.

Remember to use the OPA only in the unresponsive patient with *no cough or gag reflex.* If the patient has a cough or gag reflex, the OPA may stimulate vomiting and laryngospasm.

Basic Airway Adjuncts: Nasopharyngeal Airway

Introduction

The nasopharyngeal airway (NPA) is used as an alternative to an OPA in patients who need a basic airway management adjunct. The NPA is a soft rubber or plastic uncuffed tube (Figure 3A) that provides a conduit for airflow between the nares and the pharynx.

Unlike oral airways, NPAs *may be used in conscious or semiconscious patients* (patients with an intact cough and gag reflex). The NPA is indicated when insertion of an OPA is technically difficult or impossible. Examples include patients with a strong gag reflex, trismus, massive trauma around the mouth, or wiring of the jaws. The NPA may also be used in patients who are neurologically impaired with poor pharyngeal tone or coordination leading to upper airway obstruction.

Technique of NPA Insertion

Step	Action
1	**Select the proper size NPA.** • Compare the outer circumference of the NPA with the inner aperture of the nares. The NPA should not be so large that it causes sustained blanching of the nostrils. Some providers use the diameter of the patient's smallest finger as a guide to selecting the proper size. • The length of the NPA should be the same as the distance from the tip of the patient's nose to the earlobe.
2	**Lubricate the airway** with a water-soluble lubricant or anesthetic jelly.
3	**Insert the airway** through the nostril in a posterior direction perpendicular to the plane of the face. Pass it gently along the floor of the nasopharynx (Figure 3B). If you encounter resistance: • Slightly rotate the tube to facilitate insertion at the angle of the nasal passage and nasopharynx • Attempt placement through the other nostril because patients have different-sized nasal passages

Reevaluate frequently. Maintain head tilt by providing anterior displacement of the mandible using chin lift or jaw thrust. Mucus, blood, vomit, or the soft tissues of the pharynx can obstruct the NPA, which has a small internal diameter. *Frequent evaluation and suctioning of the airway may be necessary to ensure patency.*

Cautions

Be aware of the following when using an NPA:

• Take care to insert the airway gently to avoid complications. The airway can irritate the mucosa or lacerate adenoidal tissue and cause bleeding, with possible aspiration of clots into the trachea. Suction may be necessary to remove blood or secretions.

• An improperly sized NPA may enter the esophagus. With active ventilation, such as bag-mask, the NPA may cause gastric inflation and possible hypoventilation.

• An NPA may cause laryngospasm and vomiting, even though it is commonly tolerated by semiconscious patients.

• Use caution in patients with facial trauma because of the risk of misplacement into the cranial cavity thorough a fractured cribiform plate.

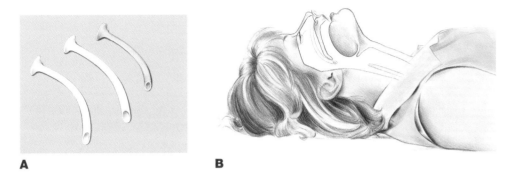

Figure 3. Nasopharyngeal airways. **A**, Three nasopharyngeal airway devices. **B**, One nasopharyngeal airway device inserted.

Foundation Facts: **Precautions for OPAs and NPAs**	Take the following precautions when using an OPA or NPA: • Always check spontaneous respirations immediately after insertion of either an OPA or NPA. • If respirations are absent or inadequate, start positive-pressure ventilations at once with an appropriate device. • If adjuncts are unavailable, use mouth-to-mask barrier ventilation.

Suctioning

Introduction

Suctioning is an essential component of maintaining a patient's airway. Providers should be prepared to perform suctioning immediately if the airway becomes occluded with secretions, blood, or vomit.

Suction devices consist of both portable and wall-mounted units.

- Portable suction devices are easy to transport but may not provide adequate suction power. A suction force of -80 to -120 mm Hg is generally necessary.
- Wall-mounted suction units should be capable of providing a vacuum of more than -300 mm Hg when the tube is clamped at full suction.

Soft vs Rigid Catheters

Both soft flexible and rigid suctioning catheters are available.

Soft flexible catheters may be used in the mouth or nose. Soft flexible catheters are available in sterile wrappers and can also be used for ET tube deep suctioning.

Rigid catheters (eg, Yankauer) are used to suction the oropharynx. These are better for suctioning thick secretions and particulate matter.

Catheter type	Use for
Soft	• Aspiration of thin secretions from the oropharynx and naso-pharynx • Performing intratracheal suctioning • Suctioning through an in-place airway (ie, NPA) to access the back of the pharynx in a patient with clenched teeth
Rigid	• More effective suctioning of the oropharynx, particularly if there is thick particulate matter

Oropharyngeal Suctioning Procedure

Follow the steps below to perform oropharyngeal suctioning.

Step	Action
1	Gently insert the suction catheter or device into the oropharynx beyond the tongue. Measure the catheter before suctioning, and do not insert it any further than the distance from the tip of the nose to the earlobe.
2	Apply suction by occluding the side opening while withdrawing the catheter with a rotating or twisting motion. **Typically limit suction attempts to 10 seconds or less.** To avoid hypoxemia precede and follow suctioning attempts with a short period of administration of 100% oxygen.

Monitor the patient's heart rate, pulse, oxygen saturation, and clinical appearance during suctioning. If bradycardia develops or clinical appearance deteriorates, interrupt suctioning. Administer a high oxygen concentration until the heart rate returns to normal.

Endotracheal Tube Suctioning Procedure

Patients with pulmonary secretions may require suctioning even after endotracheal intubation. Follow the steps below to perform ET tube suctioning:

Step	Action
1	Use sterile technique to reduce the likelihood of airway contamination.
2	Gently insert the catheter into the ET tube. Be sure the side opening is not occluded during insertion. Insertion of the catheter beyond the tip of the ET tube is not recommended because it may injure the endotracheal mucosa or stimulate coughing or bronchospasm.
3	Apply suction by occluding the side opening only while withdrawing the catheter with a rotating or twisting motion. **Suction attempts should not exceed 10 seconds.** To avoid hypoxemia, precede and follow suctioning attempts with a short period of administration of 100% oxygen. To help remove thick mucus or other material from the airway, instill 1 or 2 mL of sterile saline into the airway before suctioning. Provide positive-pressure ventilation to disperse the saline throughout the airways for maximum effect.

Monitor the patient's heart rate, pulse, oxygen saturation, and clinical appearance during suctioning. If bradycardia develops, oxygen saturation drops, or clinical appearance deteriorates, interrupt suctioning at once. Administer high-flow oxygen until the heart rate returns to normal and the clinical condition improves. Assist ventilation as needed.

Providing Ventilation With an Advanced Airway

Introduction

Selection of an advanced airway device depends on the training, scope of practice, and equipment of the providers on the resuscitation team. Advanced airways include

- Combitube
- LMA
- ET tube

Because a small proportion of patients cannot be ventilated with an LMA, providers who use this device should have an alternative airway management strategy. A bag-mask can be this alternate strategy.

This course will familiarize you with types of advanced airways. Instruction in the skilled placement of these airways is beyond the scope of the basic ACLS Provider Course. To be proficient in the use of advanced airway devices, you must have adequate initial training and ongoing experience. Providers who insert advanced airways must participate in a process of continuous quality improvement to document and minimize complications.

In this course you will practice ventilating with an advanced airway in place and integrating ventilation with chest compressions.

Combitube

The Combitube is an advanced airway alternative to endotracheal intubation. This device provides adequate ventilation comparable to an ET tube. It is acceptable to use the Combitube as an alternative to an ET tube for airway management in cardiac arrest. Fatal complications may occur with use of the Combitube. Only providers experienced with its use should perform Combitube insertion.

See the student CD for more information on the Combitube.

LMA

The laryngeal mask airway (LMA) is another advanced airway alternative to endotracheal intubation and provides comparable ventilation. As with the Combitube, it is acceptable to use the LMA as an alternative to an ET tube for airway management in cardiac arrest. Only experienced providers should perform LMA insertion.

See the student CD for more information on the LMA.

Endotracheal Intubation

Only experienced providers should perform endotracheal intubation. See the Endotracheal Intubation section on the student CD for more information on this procedure.

A brief summary of the basic steps for performing endotracheal intubation are given here to familiarize the ACLS provider who may assist with the procedure.

- Prepare for intubation by assembling the necessary equipment.
- Ask another team member to apply *cricoid pressure* if the patient is unconscious with no cough or gag reflex.
- Perform endotracheal intubation (see the student CD).
- Inflate cuff or cuffs on the tube.
- Attach the ventilation bag
- Confirm correct placement by physical examination and a confirmation device (eg, exhaled CO_2 detector or esophageal detector device).
- Secure the tube in place.
- Monitor for displacement.

Cricoid Pressure

Use cricoid pressure only during insertion of an ET tube and only if the patient is deeply unconscious—no gag or cough reflexes.

During insertion of an ET tube in adults, one provider may apply *cricoid pressure* while another performs the procedure. This pressure may help minimize regurgitation of gastric contents and may facilitate tube placement through the tracheal orifice. Maintain cricoid pressure until the advanced airway cuff is inflated and proper tube position has been confirmed. Application of cricoid pressure during cardiac arrest usually requires a third rescuer who is not responsible for compressions or ventilation.

See the student CD for specific cricoid pressure techniques.

Foundation Facts:

Rescue Breaths for CPR With an Advanced Airway in Place

Rescue Breathing Without an Advanced Airway and Without Chest Compressions

During CPR the compression-to-ventilation ratio is 30:2. But once an advanced airway is in place (ie, ET tube, Combitube, or LMA), chest compressions are no longer interrupted for ventilations.

With an advanced airway in place, give 1 breath every 6 to 8 seconds (approximately 8 to 10 breaths per minute) without trying to synchronize breaths between compressions. Ideally the breath should be given during chest recoil between chest compressions. Continuously reevaluate compressions and ventilations. Modifications may be necessary if either is ineffective.

In this case the patient has a pulse and compressions are not indicated. Give one ventilation every 5 to 6 seconds or approximately 10 to 12 breaths per minute.

Precautions for Trauma Patients

Summary

When providing assisted ventilation for patients with known or suspected cervical spine trauma, avoid unnecessary spine movement. Excessive head and neck movement in patients with an unstable cervical spinal column can cause irreversible injury to the spinal cord or worsen a minor spinal cord injury. Approximately 2% of patients with blunt trauma serious enough to require spinal imaging in the ED have a spinal injury. This risk is tripled if the patient has a head or facial injury. Assume that any patient with multiple traumas, head injury, or facial trauma has a spine injury. Be particularly cautious if a patient has suspected cervical spine injury. Examples are patients who have experienced a high-speed motor vehicle collision, have fallen from a height, or have been injured while diving.

Follow these precautions if cervical spine trauma is suspected:

- Open the airway using a jaw thrust *without head extension*. Because maintaining a patent airway and providing adequate ventilation are priorities, use a head tilt–chin lift maneuver if the jaw thrust is not effective.

- Have another team member stabilize the head in a neutral position during all airway manipulation. **Use manual spinal motion restriction rather than immobilization devices.** Manual spinal immobilization is safer. Cervical collars may complicate airway management. Immobilization devices may interfere with airway patency. Cervical collars may increase intracranial pressure in patients with head trauma.

- Use spinal immobilization devices, however, during transport.

VF Treated With CPR and AED Case

Introduction	This case will prepare you with the knowledge you need to pass the CPR/AED testing station. This case discusses how to respond as a lone rescuer to an out-of-hospital emergency, equipped with only CPR skills and an automated external defibrillator (AED). The case scenario presents a *patient who collapses from either VF or VT.* The only equipment available is an AED stocked with a pocket face mask. Because other rescuers are not present, you must care for the patient without help.

ACLS interventions, including advanced airway control and IV medications, are not options in this scenario.

Note that during the course you will be required to demonstrate both your knowledge of this case and competency in basic skill performance. |
| ***Learning Objectives*** | By the end of this case you should be able to

1. Recognize a patient who may be in VF/pulseless VT
2. Implement the BLS Healthcare Provider Algorithm, perform 1-rescuer CPR, and operate an AED |
| ***Rhythms for VF Treated With CPR and an AED*** | With an AED there are no rhythms to learn. The AED will answer the question:

• Is the rhythm shockable, ie, VF or pulseless VT? |
| ***Drugs for VF Treated With CPR and an AED*** | There are no new drugs to learn in this case. You will use only your CPR skills and an AED. |

BLS Primary Survey

Introduction	The BLS Primary Survey is used in all cases of cardiac arrest. The first steps in the treatment of any emergency are to *check patient responsiveness, activate EMS,* and *get the AED.* Then you perform the ABCDs.

In the respiratory arrest case you learned the basics of airway assessment and management of a patient in respiratory arrest with a pulse. In this case you will assess and manage a patient without a pulse and use the AED. |

**Airway
Breathing
Circulation**

Perform these BLS Primary Survey steps:

Airway	• While observing the patient's chest: Look for the chest to rise and fall. Listen for air escaping during exhalation. Feel for the flow of air against your cheek. • Open the airway using noninvasive techniques (head tilt–chin lift or jaw thrust without head extension if trauma is suspected).
Breathing	Check breathing (take at least 5 seconds and no more than 10 seconds). If breathing is not adequate give 2 rescue breaths. Use a barrier device if available. Give each breath over 1 second. Each breath should make the chest rise. Do not ventilate too fast (rate) or too much (volume).
Circulation	• Check the patient's carotid pulse (take at least 5 seconds and not more than 10 seconds). • If you do not definitely feel a pulse, perform cycles of compressions and ventilations (30:2 ratio) until an AED arrives. • Perform chest compressions at a depth of 1½ to 2 inches. Push hard and fast at a rate of 100 compressions per minute. Allow complete chest recoil. *Perform high-quality CPR until an AED arrives and pads are placed and the AED is ready to analyze the patient.*
Defibrillation (Using an AED)	• Attach the AED. • Follow AED prompts. • Follow each shock immediately with CPR, beginning with chest compressions.

Foundation Facts:

Starting CPR When You Are Not Sure About Pulse

If you are not sure whether the patient has a pulse, you should begin cycles of compressions and ventilations. Unnecessary compressions are less harmful than failing to provide necessary compressions when they are needed. CPR in the patient with a pulse is not harmful. Delaying or failing to start CPR in a patient without a pulse reduces the chance of a successful resuscitation.

Purpose of Defibrillation

Defibrillation does not restart the heart. Defibrillation stuns the heart and briefly terminates all electrical activity, including VF and rapid VT. If the heart is still viable, its normal pacemakers may eventually resume electrical activity (return of spontaneous rhythm) that ultimately results in a perfusing rhythm.

In the first minutes after successful defibrillation, however, any spontaneous rhythm is typically slow and does not create pulses or perfusion. CPR is needed for several minutes until adequate heart function resumes. This is the rationale for resuming immediate high-quality chest compressions after a shock.

Principle of Early Defibrillation

The interval from collapse to defibrillation is one of the most important determinants of survival from cardiac arrest. Early defibrillation is critical for victims of sudden cardiac arrest for the following reasons:

- The most common initial rhythms in witnessed sudden cardiac arrest are VF or rapid, pulseless VT. Pulseless VT rapidly deteriorates to VF. When VF is present, the heart quivers and does not pump blood.
- The only effective treatment for VF is electrical defibrillation (delivery of a shock to stop the VF).
- The probability of successful defibrillation decreases quickly over time.
- VF deteriorates to asystole if not treated.

The earlier defibrillation occurs, the higher the survival rate. When VF is present, CPR can provide a small amount of blood flow to the heart and brain but cannot directly restore an organized rhythm. Restoration of a perfusing rhythm requires immediate CPR and defibrillation within a few minutes of the initial arrest.

For every minute that passes between collapse and defibrillation, the chance of survival from a witnessed VF sudden cardiac arrest (SCA) declines by 7% to 10% per minute if no bystander CPR is provided. When bystander CPR is given the decline is more gradual and averages 3% to 4% per minute from collapse to defibrillation. CPR can double or triple survival from witnessed SCA at most defibrillation intervals. See Figures 4 and 5.

Lay rescuer AED programs increase the likelihood that people (lay rescuers and healthcare providers) who can perform CPR and attempt defibrillation will be available. This helps shorten the time between collapse and defibrillation for a greater number of victims of sudden cardiac arrest.

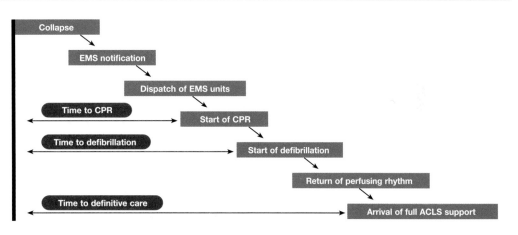

Figure 4. Sequence of events and key intervals that occur with cardiac arrest.

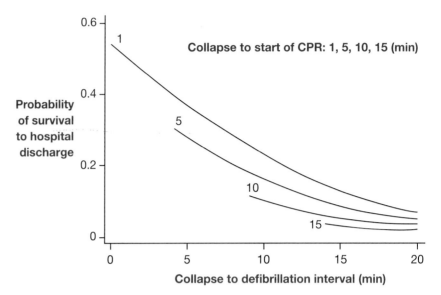

Figure 5. Effect of collapse-to-CPR interval and collapse-to-defibrillation interval on survival to hospital discharge. The graph displays the probability of survival to hospital discharge in relation to 4 intervals from collapse to start of CPR (1, 5, 10, and 15 minutes) and collapse to defibrillation (5, 10, 15, and 20 minutes). To determine the probability of survival for an individual patient, identify the curve indicating the interval between collapse and CPR, and then identify the point on that curve that corresponds to the interval from collapse to defibrillation (see horizontal axis). The probability of survival is then indicated on the vertical axis. Based on data from King County, Washington (N=1667 witnessed VT/VF arrests), with additional cases from Tucson, Arizona (N=205 witnessed VT/VF arrests).

AED Operation

Use AEDs only when patients have the following 3 clinical findings:

- No response
- No breathing
- No pulse

The patient in cardiac arrest may demonstrate agonal gasps. Agonal gasps may happen in the first minutes after sudden cardiac arrest. Agonal gasps are *not* adequate breathing. A patient who has agonal gasps, does not respond, and has no pulse is in cardiac arrest.

Critical Concepts:
Agonal Gasps

Remember that agonal gasps are not adequate breathing.

Know Your AED

You must know the AED used in your clinical setting and be ready to use it at any time. Review the troubleshooting checklist supplied by the AED manufacturer. Learn to perform daily maintenance checks. Not only are these checks an effective review of the steps of operation, but also they are a means of verifying that the AED is ready for use.

See the student CD for a sample "readiness-for-use" AED checklist.

The Universal AED: Common Steps to Operate All AEDs

Once the AED arrives, put it at the patient's side, next to the rescuer who will operate it. This position provides ready access to the AED controls and easy placement of electrode pads. It also allows a second rescuer to perform CPR from the opposite side of the patient without interfering with AED operation.

AEDs are available in different models. Although there are small differences from model to model, all AEDs operate in basically the same way. The following table lists the 4 universal steps for operating an AED:

Step	Action
1	**POWER ON the AED** (this activates voice prompts for guidance in all subsequent steps). • Open the carrying case or the top of the AED. • Turn the power on (some devices will "power on" automatically when you open the lid or case).
2	**ATTACH ELECTRODE PADS** to the patient's bare chest. • Choose correct pads (adult vs child) for size/age of the patient. Use child pads or a child system for children less than 8 years of age if available. ***Do not use child pads or a child system for patients 8 years and older.*** • Peel the backing away from the electrode pads. • Quickly wipe the patient's chest if it is covered with water or sweat. • Attach the adhesive electrode pads to the patient's bare chest. — Place one electrode pad on the upper-right side of the bare chest to the right of the breastbone directly below the collarbone. — Place the other pad to the left of the nipple, with the top margin of the pad a few inches below the left armpit (Figure 6). • Attach the AED connecting cables to the AED box (some are preconnected).
3	**ANALYZE THE RHYTHM.** • Always clear the patient during analysis. Be sure no one is touching the victim, not even the person in charge of giving breaths. • Some AEDs will instruct you to push a button to allow the AED to begin analyzing the heart rhythm; others will do that automatically. The AED rhythm analysis may take about 5 to 15 seconds. • The AED then instructs whether or not a shock is needed.
4	If the AED advises a shock, it will tell you to **BE SURE TO CLEAR THE PATIENT.** • Clear the patient before delivering the shock; be sure no one is touching the patient. • Loudly state a "clear the patient" message, such as "I'm clear, you're clear, everybody's clear" or simply "Clear." • Perform a visual check to ensure that no one is in contact with the patient. • Press the **SHOCK** button. • The shock will produce a sudden contraction of the patient's muscles.

As soon as the shock is delivered, resume CPR, starting with chest compressions, with cycles of compressions and breaths at a 30:2 ratio. Do not perform a pulse or rhythm check. After 2 minutes of CPR, the AED will prompt you to repeat steps 3 and 4.

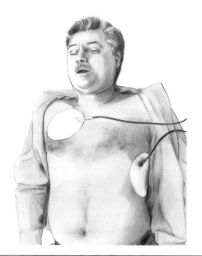

Figure 6. AED electrode pad placement on the patient.

Troubleshooting the AED

Studies of AED "failures" have shown that most problems are caused by operator error rather than by AED defects. Operator error is less likely if the operator is experienced in using the AED, has had recurrent training or practice with the AED, and is using an AED that has been well maintained.

If the AED does not promptly analyze the rhythm, do the following:

- Resume high-quality chest compressions and ventilations.
- Check all connections between the AED and the patient to make sure that they are intact.

> *Never delay chest compressions to troubleshoot the AED.*

Shock First vs CPR First

When you care for an unresponsive, nonbreathing, pulseless adult patient, should you attempt to shock first with an AED or provide CPR first? The following points address this issue:

- When you witness an out-of-hospital adult arrest and an AED is available, use the AED as soon as possible. You may perform chest compressions until the AED has been applied and is ready for rhythm analysis.
- Healthcare providers who treat cardiac arrest in the hospital and other facilities with an AED should provide immediate CPR, then use the AED as soon as it is available.
- EMS system medical directors may consider following a protocol that allows EMS responders to give 2 minutes (about 5 cycles) of CPR before attempting defibrillation with an AED, particularly when the call-to-response time interval is longer than 4 to 5 minutes or if they did not witness the arrest.
- Follow the AED voice prompts. The AED will analyze the heart rhythm and, if indicated, instruct you to deliver a shock. If the rhythm that is detected is nonshockable, the AED will instruct you to resume CPR immediately, starting with chest compressions.
- Remember to minimize interruptions in chest compressions.

AED Use in Special Situations

Introduction

The following special situations may require the operator to take extra care in placing the electrode pads when using an AED:

- The patient has a hairy chest.
- The patient is immersed in water or water is covering the patient's chest.
- The patient has an implanted pacemaker or defibrillator.
- The patient has a transdermal medication patch or other object on the surface of the skin where the AED electrode pads are placed.

Hairy Chest

If the patient has a hairy chest, the AED pads may stick to the hair and may not stick to the skin on the chest. If this occurs, the AED will not be able to analyze the patient's heart rhythm. The AED will give a "check electrodes" or "check electrode pads" message. If this happens complete the following steps and actions without (or with minimal) interruption in chest compressions.

Step	Action
1	If the pads stick to the hair instead of the skin, press down firmly on each pad.
2	If the AED continues to prompt you to "check pads" or "check electrodes," quickly pull off the pads. This will remove much of the hair.
3	If too much hair still remains where you will put the pads, shave the area with the razor in the AED carrying case if available.
4	Put on a new set of pads. Follow the AED voice prompts.

Water

Water conducts electricity. Do not use an AED in the water. If the patient's chest is covered with water, water may conduct the shock electricity across the skin of the chest. This will prevent the delivery of an adequate shock dose to the heart.

Handle these situations as follows:

If...	Then...
The patient is in the water	Pull the patient out of the water
The patient's chest is covered with water	Wipe the chest quickly before attaching the electrodes
The patient is lying on snow or in a small puddle	Use the AED

Implanted Pacemaker

Patients who are known to be at high risk for sudden cardiac arrest may have implanted defibrillators/pacemakers that deliver shocks directly to the heart muscle. You can immediately identify these devices because they create a hard lump beneath the skin of the upper chest or abdomen. The lump is half the size of a deck of cards, with a small overlying scar. The presence of an implanted defibrillator or pacemaker is not a contraindication to applying and using an AED as long as you do not place the AED electrode pads directly over the device. The reason to avoid placing an AED electrode pad directly over an implanted medical device is that the device may block delivery of the shock to the heart.

If you identify an implanted defibrillator/pacemaker:

- Place the AED electrode pad at least 1 inch (2.5 cm) to either side of the implanted device
- Follow the normal steps for operating an AED

Occasionally the analysis and shock cycles of implanted defibrillators and AEDs will conflict. If the implanted defibrillator is delivering shocks to the patient (the patient's muscles contract in a manner like that observed after an AED shock), allow 30 to 60 seconds for the implanted defibrillator to complete the treatment cycle before delivering a shock from the AED.

Transdermal Medication Patches

Do not place AED electrodes directly on top of a medication patch (eg, a patch of nitroglycerin, nicotine, pain medication, hormone replacement therapy, or antihypertensive medication). The medication patch may block the transfer of energy from the electrode pad to the heart, and the delivery of a shock through the patch may also cause small burns to the skin. To prevent the medication patch from blocking delivery of energy, remove the patch and wipe the area clean before attaching the AED electrode pad. Try to minimize interruptions in chest compressions.

VF/Pulseless VT Case
Persistent/Refractory/Recurrent and Shock Resistant

Introduction

This case focuses on the assessment and actions used for a *witnessed cardiac arrest due to ventricular fibrillation (VF) or pulseless ventricular tachycardia (VT) that is resistant (unresponsive) to the first shock.* You will use a manual defibrillator in this case.

In this case and the course you will have an opportunity to demonstrate effective resuscitation team behaviors while performing the assessment and action skills typically used within the first 10 minutes of a cardiac arrest. During the BLS Primary Survey, team members will perform continuous high-quality CPR with effective chest compressions and ventilation with a bag-mask device. The team leader will conduct the ACLS Secondary Survey, including rhythm recognition (shockable versus nonshockable), defibrillation using a manual defibrillator, resuscitation drugs, a discussion of IV/IO access, and advanced airways.

Remember that the success of any resuscitation attempt is built on a strong base of high-quality CPR and defibrillation when required by the patient's ECG rhythm.

Learning Objectives

By the end of this case you will be able to

1. Recognize VF and VT on the ECG
2. Manage VF/pulseless VT according to the ACLS Pulseless Arrest Algorithm
3. Recall indications, contraindications, doses, and routes of administration for drugs recommended for refractory VF/pulseless VT
4. Perform defibrillation with minimal interruption of chest compressions
5. Coordinate team functions while ensuring continuous high-quality CPR, defibrillation, and rhythm assessment

Rhythms for VF/ Pulseless VT	This case involves these ECG rhythms:

- VF
- VT
- ECG artifact that looks like VF

Drugs for VF/Pulseless VT	This case involves these drugs:

- Epinephrine
- Vasopressin
- Amiodarone
- Lidocaine
- Magnesium sulfate

Managing VF/Pulseless VT: The ACLS Pulseless Arrest Algorithm

Overview

The ACLS Pulseless Arrest Algorithm (Figure 7) is the most important algorithm to know for adult resuscitation. This algorithm outlines all the steps for assessment and management of the pulseless patient who does not initially respond to BLS interventions, including a first shock from an AED. In previous editions of the ECC guidelines, several algorithms were used for the pulseless arrest patient (VF/VT, asystole, PEA). Now all steps in the assessment and management of the pulseless patient appear in a single algorithm, the ACLS Pulseless Arrest Algorithm, which is easier to use and remember. The algorithm consists of the 2 pathways for a pulseless arrest:

- A shockable rhythm (VF/VT) displayed on the left side of the algorithm
- A rhythm that is nonshockable (asystole/PEA) displayed on the right side of the algorithm

Throughout the case discussion of the Pulseless Arrest Algorithm, we will refer to box numbers 1 through 13. These are the numbers assigned to the boxes on the algorithm.

VF/VT (Left Side)

Because many patients of sudden cardiac arrest demonstrate VF at some point in their arrest, it is expected that ACLS providers will frequently follow the left side of the ACLS Pulseless Arrest Algorithm (Figure 7). Rapid treatment of VF according to this sequence is the best scientific approach to restoring spontaneous circulation.

Pulseless VT is included in the algorithm because it is treated as VF. VF and pulseless VT require CPR until a defibrillator is available. Both are treated with high-energy unsynchronized shocks.

Asystole/PEA (Right Side)

The right side of the algorithm outlines the sequence of actions to perform if the rhythm is nonshockable. You will have an opportunity to practice this sequence in the asystole and PEA cases.

Summary

The VF/pulseless VT case gives you an opportunity to practice performing rapid treatment of VF/VT following the steps on the left side of the ACLS Pulseless Arrest Algorithm (Boxes 1 through 8).

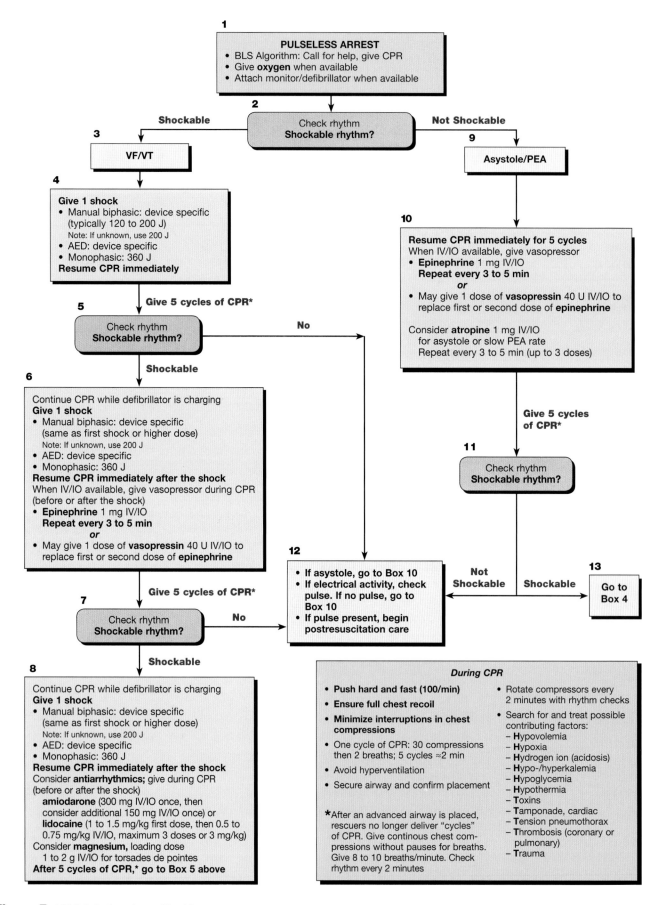

1

PULSELESS ARREST
- BLS Algorithm: Call for help, give CPR
- Give **oxygen** when available
- Attach monitor/defibrillator when available

2 Check rhythm
Shockable rhythm?

Shockable ← → **Not Shockable**

3 VF/VT

9 Asystole/PEA

4
Give 1 shock
- Manual biphasic: device specific (typically 120 to 200 J)
  Note: If unknown, use 200 J
- AED: device specific
- Monophasic: 360 J
Resume CPR immediately

Give 5 cycles of CPR*

5 Check rhythm
Shockable rhythm?

No →

Shockable

10
Resume CPR immediately for 5 cycles
When IV/IO available, give vasopressor
- **Epinephrine** 1 mg IV/IO
  Repeat every 3 to 5 min
  or
- May give 1 dose of **vasopressin** 40 U IV/IO to replace first or second dose of **epinephrine**

Consider **atropine** 1 mg IV/IO
for asystole or slow PEA rate
Repeat every 3 to 5 min (up to 3 doses)

6
Continue CPR while defibrillator is charging
Give 1 shock
- Manual biphasic: device specific (same as first shock or higher dose)
  Note: If unknown, use 200 J
- AED: device specific
- Monophasic: 360 J
Resume CPR immediately after the shock
When IV/IO available, give vasopressor during CPR (before or after the shock)
- **Epinephrine** 1 mg IV/IO
  Repeat every 3 to 5 min
  or
- May give 1 dose of **vasopressin** 40 U IV/IO to replace first or second dose of **epinephrine**

Give 5 cycles of CPR*

7 Check rhythm
Shockable rhythm?

No →

Shockable

Give 5 cycles of CPR*

11 Check rhythm
Shockable rhythm?

12
- If asystole, go to Box 10
- If electrical activity, check pulse. If no pulse, go to Box 10
- If pulse present, begin postresuscitation care

Not Shockable | **Shockable**

13 Go to Box 4

8
Continue CPR while defibrillator is charging
Give 1 shock
- Manual biphasic: device specific (same as first shock or higher dose)
  Note: If unknown, use 200 J
- AED: device specific
- Monophasic: 360 J
Resume CPR immediately after the shock
Consider **antiarrhythmics;** give during CPR (before or after the shock)
  amiodarone (300 mg IV/IO once, then consider additional 150 mg IV/IO once) or
  lidocaine (1 to 1.5 mg/kg first dose, then 0.5 to 0.75 mg/kg IV/IO, maximum 3 doses or 3 mg/kg)
Consider **magnesium,** loading dose 1 to 2 g IV/IO for torsades de pointes
After 5 cycles of CPR,* go to Box 5 above

During CPR
- **Push hard and fast (100/min)**
- **Ensure full chest recoil**
- **Minimize interruptions in chest compressions**
- One cycle of CPR: 30 compressions then 2 breaths; 5 cycles ≈2 min
- Avoid hyperventilation
- Secure airway and confirm placement

*After an advanced airway is placed, rescuers no longer deliver "cycles" of CPR. Give continous chest compressions without pauses for breaths. Give 8 to 10 breaths/minute. Check rhythm every 2 minutes

- Rotate compressors every 2 minutes with rhythm checks
- Search for and treat possible contributing factors:
  – **H**ypovolemia
  – **H**ypoxia
  – **H**ydrogen ion (acidosis)
  – **H**ypo-/hyperkalemia
  – **H**ypoglycemia
  – **H**ypothermia
  – **T**oxins
  – **T**amponade, cardiac
  – **T**ension pneumothorax
  – **T**hrombosis (coronary or pulmonary)
  – **T**rauma

Figure 7. ACLS Pulseless Arrest Algorithm.

Application of the Pulseless Arrest Algorithm—VF/VT Pathway

Introduction
(Boxes 1-4)

This case discusses the assessment and treatment of a patient with refractory VF or pulseless VT. At this point in the algorithm, the BLS Primary Survey has already been conducted, including activation of the emergency response system, performing CPR, attaching the manual defibrillator, and delivering the first shock (boxes 1 through 4).

The ACLS resuscitation team now intervenes and conducts the ACLS Secondary Survey. In this case the secondary **ABCDs** are assessed and actions taken as needed. The team leader coordinates the efforts of the resuscitation team in the performance of the steps listed on the VF/VT pathway on the left side of the Pulseless Arrest Algorithm.

Minimal Interruption of Chest Compressions

A team member should continue to perform high-quality CPR until the defibrillator arrives and is attached to the patient. The team leader assigns roles and responsibilities and organizes interventions to minimize interruptions in chest compressions. This accomplishes the most critical interventions for VF or pulseless VT: CPR with minimal interruptions in chest compressions and defibrillation during the first minutes of arrest.

Continued use of an AED (or the automatic mode) is not recommended when a manual defibrillator is present and the provider skills are adequate for rhythm interpretation. Use of an AED may result in unnecessarily prolonged interruptions in chest compressions for rhythm analysis and shock administration.

> *Chest compressions should ideally be interrupted only for ventilation (unless an advanced airway is placed), rhythm checks, and actual shock delivery.*

Foundation Facts:

Resume CPR While Manual Defibrillator Is Charging

Resume CPR while the manual defibrillator is charging if charging takes more than 10 seconds. Even a 5- to 10-second pause in chest compressions reduces the chance that a shock will terminate VF. For an AED, follow the manufacturer's prompts.

New-model manual defibrillators charge rapidly (<10 seconds), so that chest compressions during charge are unnecessary. Older-model manual defibrillators may take longer to charge, so chest compressions during charging are advised to minimize time between last compression and shock delivery. You should know your manual defibrillator charge time and whether compressions during charging are needed.

Deliver 1 Shock
(Box 4)

Box 4 directs the delivery of 1 shock. Note the change from previous guidelines, which recommended up to 3 shocks. The energy dose used is determined by whether the defibrillator is monophasic or biphasic.

CPR is immediately resumed, beginning with chest compressions. A rhythm or pulse check is not performed.

If you are using a *monophasic* defibrillator, give a single 360-J shock. Use the same energy dose for subsequent shocks.

Biphasic defibrillators use a variety of waveforms, each of which is effective for terminating VF over a specific dose range. It is reasonable to use selected energies of 150 J to 200 J with a biphasic truncated exponential waveform or 120 J with a rectilinear waveform for the initial shock.

The biphasic defibrillator manufacturer should display the effective biphasic waveform dose range on the face of the device. If you do not know the effective biphasic dose range of the device, deliver 200 J for the first shock and an equal or higher dose for subsequent shocks. The 200-J default energy level was chosen because it falls within the reported range of doses effective for first and subsequent biphasic shocks. This energy level can be provided by every biphasic manual defibrillator available when the *2005 AHA Guidelines for CPR and ECC* were published.

If VF is initially terminated by a shock but recurs later in the resuscitation attempt, deliver subsequent shocks at the previously successful energy level.

> *Immediately after the shock, resume CPR, beginning with chest compressions. Give 2 minutes (about 5 cycles) of CPR. A cycle consists of 30 compressions followed by 2 ventilations in the patient without an advanced airway.*

Foundation Facts:

Clearing for Defibrillation

To ensure safety during defibrillation, always announce when you are about to deliver a shock. State a "warning" firmly and in a forceful voice before delivering each shock (this entire sequence should take less than 5 seconds):

- **"I am going to shock on three. One, I'm clear."** Check to make sure you are clear of contact with the patient, the stretcher, or other equipment.

- **"Two, you're clear."** Make a visual check to ensure that no one is touching the patient or stretcher. In particular, check the person providing ventilations. That person's hands should not be touching the ventilatory adjuncts, including an advanced airway. Be sure oxygen is not flowing across the patient's chest. Turn oxygen off or direct flow away from the patient's chest. Ideally, make sure the source of oxygen is removed from the patient when you clear the patient to shock.

- **"Three, everybody is clear."** Check yourself one more time before pressing the SHOCK button.

You need not use these exact words, but you must warn others that you are about to deliver shocks and that everyone must stand clear.

Rhythm Check (Box 5)

Box 5 directs you to conduct a rhythm check after 2 minutes (about 5 cycles) of CPR. Be careful to minimize interruptions in chest compressions.

> *The pause in chest compressions to check the rhythm should ideally not exceed 10 seconds.*

If a nonshockable rhythm is present and the rhythm is organized (complexes appear regular and narrow), a team member should try to palpate a pulse. Remember, rhythm and pulse checks should be brief (not more than 10 seconds). *Perform a pulse check—preferably during rhythm analysis—only if an organized rhythm is present.* Remember, take no more than 10 seconds to perform a rhythm analysis or pulse check. If there is any doubt about the presence of a pulse, immediately resume CPR.

If the rhythm check reveals a nonshockable rhythm and there is no pulse, then proceed along the asystole/PEA pathway on the right side of the ACLS Pulseless Arrest Algorithm. If the rhythm check reveals a shockable rhythm and if appropriate for the defibrillator in use, resume CPR, beginning with chest compressions, while the defibrillator is charging. During CPR while the defibrillator is charging, pay careful attention to the safety of the team member performing chest compressions. Remember to clear before the shock!

Foundation Facts:	Conductive materials are used to reduce transthoracic impedance (resistance to the electrical current) to shocks. Conductive materials include paddles with electrode paste, gel pads, or self-adhesive pads. No existing data suggests that one is better. Use of self-adhesive pads will, however, reduce the risk of arcing. Self-adhesive pads can also be applied for monitoring, and they allow for the rapid delivery of a shock if necessary. For these reasons they are routinely recommended instead of paddles.
Paddles vs Pads	

Shock and Vasopressors (Box 6)

For persistent VF/pulseless VT give 1 shock and resume CPR immediately after the shock.

> *Immediately after the shock, resume CPR, beginning with chest compressions. Give 2 minutes (about 5 cycles) of CPR. A cycle consists of 30 compressions followed by 2 ventilations in the patient without an advanced airway.*

When IV/IO access is available, give a vasopressor during CPR (either before or after the shock) as follows:

- **Epinephrine** 1 mg IV/IO—repeat every 3 to 5 minutes
  OR
- **Vasopressin** 40 U IV/IO—may substitute for the first or second dose of epinephrine

Note: If additional team members are available, they should anticipate the need for drugs and prepare drugs in advance.

Epinephrine hydrochloride is used during resuscitation primarily for its α-adrenergic effects, ie, vasoconstriction. Vasoconstriction increases cerebral and coronary blood flow during CPR as mean arterial pressure and aortic diastolic pressure are increased. In previous studies, escalating and high-dose epinephrine administration did not improve survival to discharge or neurologic outcome after resuscitation from cardiac arrest.

Vasopressin is a nonadrenergic peripheral vasoconstrictor. Overall, vasopressin effects have not been shown to differ from epinephrine. A meta-analysis of 5 randomized trials found no difference between vasopressin and epinephrine for ROSC, 24-hour survival, or survival to hospital discharge.

Rhythm Check (Box 7)

Box 7 directs you to conduct a rhythm check after 2 minutes (about 5 cycles) of CPR. Be careful to minimize interruptions in chest compressions.

> *Interruption in CPR to conduct a rhythm analysis ideally should not exceed 10 seconds.*

If the rhythm check reveals a nonshockable rhythm and there is no pulse, then proceed along the asystole/PEA pathway on the right side of the ACLS Pulseless Arrest Algorithm. If the rhythm check reveals a shockable rhythm, resume chest compressions if indicated while the defibrillator is charging. The team leader is responsible for team safety while compressions are being performed and the defibrillator is charging.

Shock and Antiarrhythmics (Box 8)

Give 1 shock and resume CPR immediately after the shock.

> *Immediately after the shock, resume CPR, beginning with chest compressions. Give 2 minutes (about 5 cycles) of CPR. A cycle consists of 30 compressions followed by 2 ventilations in the patient without an advanced airway.*

Consider giving antiarrhythmic drugs, either before or after the shock. Drugs to consider are
- **Amiodarone** 300 mg IV/IO once, then consider an additional 150 mg IV/IO once
  OR
- **Lidocaine** 1 to 1.5 mg/kg IV/IO first dose, then 0.5 to 0.75 mg/kg IV/IO at 5- to 10-minute intervals, to a maximum dose of 3 mg/kg
  OR
- **Magnesium** for torsades de pointes, loading dose 1 to 2 g IV/IO diluted in 10 mL of D_5W given IV/IO push, typically over 5 to 20 minutes

Pulseless Arrest Treatment Sequences

Pulseless Arrest Treatment Sequences (Figure 8) summarizes the recommended sequence of CPR, rhythm checks, shocks, and delivery of drugs based on expert consensus. The optimal number of cycles of CPR and shocks that should be given before starting pharmacologic therapy has not been determined. Note that rhythm checks and shocks are organized around 5 cycles of compressions and ventilations, or 2 minutes if a provider is timing the arrest.

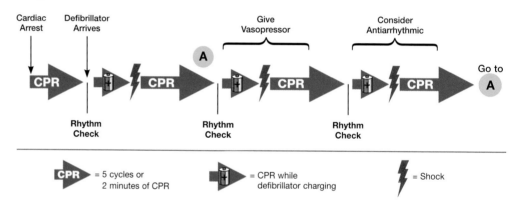

Figure 8. Pulseless Arrest: Treatment Sequences—Ventricular Fibrillation/Pulseless VT. Prepare next drug prior to rhythm check. Administer drug during CPR, as soon as possible after the rhythm check confirms VF/pulseless VT. Do not delay shock. Continue CPR while drugs are prepared and administered and defibrillator is charging. Ideally, chest compressions should be interrupted only for ventilation (until advanced airway placed), rhythm check, and actual shock delivery.

Treatment of VF/VT in Hypothermia

For a cardiac arrest patient in VF/VT who has hypothermia and a body temperature of <30°C (<86°F), a single defibrillation attempt is appropriate. If the patient fails to respond to the initial defibrillation attempt, defer subsequent defibrillation attempts and drug therapy until the core temperature rises above 30°C (86°F). The hypothermic heart may be unresponsive to drug therapy, defibrillation, and pacemaker therapy. In addition, drug metabolism is reduced. There is concern that drug levels may accumulate to toxic levels with standard dosing regimens.

For patients in moderate hypothermia (30°C to 34°C [86°F to 93.2°F]) attempt defibrillation and give medications spaced at longer intervals.

ACLS treatment of the patient with severe hypothermia, ie, core temperature less than 30°C (86°F), in cardiac arrest in the hospital should be aimed at rapid core rewarming. For more information, see the Hypothermia Algorithm in the ECC Handbook.

Resuscitation Drugs Used in VF/VT

Overview

The following classes of pharmacologic agents are used in resuscitation of VF/VT:

- Vasopressor agents: epinephrine and vasopressin
- Antiarrhythmic drugs: amiodarone, lidocaine, magnesium

Routes of access for drug administration are discussed below.

Routes of Access for Drugs

Priorities

Priorities during cardiac arrest are high-quality CPR and early defibrillation. Insertion of an advanced airway and drug administration are of secondary importance. Remember, no drug given during cardiac arrest has been shown to improve survival to hospital discharge or improve neurologic function after cardiac arrest.

Historically in ACLS, drugs have been administered either via the IV or ET route. New science and consensus opinion have reprioritized access routes. ET absorption of drugs is poor, and optimal drug dosing is not known. For this reason the IO route is preferred when IV access is not available. Priorities for vascular access are

- IV route
- IO route
- ET route

Intravenous Route

A peripheral IV is preferred for drug and fluid administration.

Central line access is not necessary during most resuscitation attempts. Central line access may cause interruptions in CPR. Alternatively, CPR can cause complications during insertion, including vascular laceration, hematomas, and bleeding. Insertion of a central noncompressible line is a relative contraindication to fibrinolytic therapy.

Establishing a peripheral line does not require interruption of CPR. Drugs, however, typically require 1 to 2 minutes to reach the central circulation when given by the IV route. Keep this in mind during the CPR sequence. The drug you give based on a rhythm check will not take effect until completion of the next cycle of CPR.

If a drug is given by the peripheral venous route, administer it as follows:

- Give the drug by bolus injection unless otherwise specified
- Follow with a 20-mL bolus of IV fluid
- Elevate the extremity for about 10 to 20 seconds to facilitate delivery of the drug to the central circulation

Intraosseous Route

Drugs and fluids during resuscitation can be delivered safely and effectively via the IO route if IV access is not available. Important points about IO access are

- IO access can be established in all age groups.
- IO access often can be achieved in 30 to 60 seconds.
- The IO route of administration is preferred over the ET route.
- Any drug or fluid that is administered IV can be given IO.

IO cannulation provides access to a noncollapsible marrow venous plexus, which serves as a rapid, safe, and reliable route for administration of drugs, crystalloids, colloids, and blood during resuscitation. The technique uses a rigid needle, preferably a specially designed IO or bone marrow needle from an IO access kit.

For more information on IO access, see the Access for Medications section on the student CD.

Endotracheal Route

IV and IO routes of administration are preferred over the ET route of administration. When considering administration of drugs via the ET route during CPR, keep these concepts in mind:

- The optimal dose of most drugs given by the ET route is unknown.
- The typical dose of drugs administered via the ET route is 2 to 2½ times the IV route.

ACLS arrest drugs that can be administered via the ET route are epinephrine, vasopressin, atropine, and lidocaine. Naloxone can also be given via the ET route. When giving drugs via the ET route, dilute the dose in 5 to 10 mL of water or normal saline. Inject the drug directly into the trachea.

Vasopressors

Introduction

There is no evidence to date that routine use of any vasopressor at any stage during management of pulseless VT, VF, or asystole increases rates of survival to hospital discharge. But there is evidence that the use of vasopressors favors initial resuscitation with ROSC.

Vasopressors Used During Cardiac Arrest

Vasopressors optimize cardiac output and blood pressure. The vasopressors used during cardiac arrest are

- Epinephrine: 1 mg IV/IO (repeat every 3 to 5 minutes)
- Vasopressin: 1 dose of 40 U IV/IO may replace either the first or second dose of epinephrine

If IV/IO access cannot be established or is delayed, give epinephrine 1:1000, 2 to 2.5 mg diluted in 5 to 10 mL of water or normal saline and injected directly into the ET tube. Remember, the ET route of drug administration results in variable and unpredictable drug absorption and blood levels.

FYI	Recent animal studies have shown that lower epinephrine concentrations achieved by the ET route may produce transient β-adrenergic effects (vasodilator effect). These β-adrenergic effects may potentially be detrimental by causing hypotension in patients with a perfusing rhythm and decreased coronary perfusion pressures during an arrest. The ACLS recommendations for ET drug dose have not changed. But the preference for IO over ET administration is emphasized.

Epinephrine

Although epinephrine has been used for years in resuscitation, there is little data to show that it improves outcome in humans. No studies have found improved rates of survival to hospital discharge or neurologic outcome when initial or escalating high-dose epinephrine was compared with standard doses. Therefore, the routine use of high-dose or escalating doses of epinephrine cannot be recommended.

Epinephrine is thought to stimulate adrenergic receptors, producing vasoconstriction, increasing blood pressure and heart rate, and improving perfusion pressure to the brain and heart.

Repeat epinephrine 1 mg IV/IO every 3 to 5 minutes during cardiac arrest.

> *Remember, follow each dose given by peripheral injection with a 20-mL flush of IV fluid and elevate the extremity above the level of the heart for 10 to 20 seconds.*

Vasopressin

Vasopressin is a nonadrenergic peripheral vasoconstrictor that causes coronary and renal vasoconstriction. Because the efficacy of vasopressin is no different than that of epinephrine in cardiac arrest, a single dose of vasopressin (40 U IV/IO) may replace either the first or second dose of epinephrine.

Antiarrhythmic Agents

Introduction

When VF/pulseless VT persists after a total of 2 or 3 shocks, separated by cycles of CPR and administration of a vasopressor, consider use of one of the following antiarrhythmics:

- Amiodarone
- Lidocaine
- Magnesium sulfate

These agents can also be used for maintenance therapy in the postresuscitation period.

Amiodarone

Consider amiodarone for treatment of VF or pulseless VT unresponsive to shock delivery, CPR, and a vasopressor. Although there is no evidence that giving any antiarrhythmic routinely during cardiac arrest increases rates of survival to hospital discharge, amiodarone has been shown to increase rates of survival to hospital admission (ie, short-term survival) compared with placebo or lidocaine.

Amiodarone is a complex drug that affects sodium, potassium, and calcium channels. It also has α-adrenergic and β-adrenergic blocking properties. Amiodarone is available in vials and prefilled syringes. During cardiac arrest consider amiodarone 300 mg IV/IO push for the first dose. If VF/pulseless VT persists, consider giving a second dose of 150 mg IV/IO in 3 to 5 minutes.

Lidocaine

Lidocaine is an alternative antiarrhythmic of long standing and widespread familiarity. However, it has no proven short-term or long-term efficacy in cardiac arrest. Lidocaine is still included as an alternative to amiodarone in settings where amiodarone is not available.

Give lidocaine in a dose of 1 to 1.5 mg/kg IV/IO. Repeat if indicated at 0.5 to 0.75 mg/kg IV/IO over 5- to 10-minute intervals to a maximum of 3 doses or 3 mg/kg. If no IV/IO access is available, then the dose for ET administration is 2 to 4 mg/kg.

Magnesium Sulfate

IV magnesium may terminate or prevent recurrent torsades de pointes in patients who have a prolonged QT interval during normal sinus rhythm. When VF/pulseless VT cardiac arrest is associated with torsades de pointes, give magnesium sulfate at a loading dose of 1 to 2 g IV/IO diluted in 10 mL D_5W given over 5 to 20 minutes. If a prearrest 12-lead ECG is available for review, check the QT interval for prolongation. Remember that pulseless VT is treated with an immediate high-energy shock, whereas magnesium is an adjunctive agent used to *prevent* recurrent or treat persistent VT associated with torsades de pointes.

Magnesium sulfate is also indicated for patients with known or suspected low serum magnesium, such as patients with alcoholism or other conditions associated with malnutrition or hypomagnesemic states. For patients in refractory VF/pulseless VT, check the patient's history, if available, for one of these conditions that suggest the presence of a reversible electrolyte abnormality.

Postresuscitation Maintenance Therapy

After conversion of VF/pulseless VT to a perfusing rhythm, consider an IV infusion of an antiarrhythmic as outlined in the table below for maintenance therapy. Usually administer the drug used or successful during the resuscitation (ie, amiodarone or lidocaine). If the patient has recurrent VF or symptomatic VT, a supplementary IV bolus of the drug if not at maximal dose or an increase in the maintenance infusion rate is usually indicated.

Agent	Dosage
Amiodarone (for recurrent VF/VT)	• Maximum cumulative dose: 2.2 g over 24 hours (based on cumulative toxicity) • Start with an IV bolus of 150 mg IV over 10 minutes • Follow by a slow infusion of 360 mg IV over the next 6 hours (1 mg/min) • Then a maintenance infusion of 540 mg IV over the next 18 hours (0.5 mg/min) **Note:** *The arrest dose is 300 mg IV/IO, repeated once if necessary at 150 mg IV/IO. If the drug has been given during cardiac arrest, start infusion as indicated. May give one 150-mg IV bolus for recurrent VF/VT; then seek expert consultation.* Monitor for hypotension bradycardia and gastrointestinal toxicity.

Agent	Dosage
Lidocaine	If the patient has not received lidocaine during the arrest: • Start with a loading dose of 1 to 1.5 mg/kg, then 0.5 to 0.75 mg/kg every 5 to 10 minutes if needed to a total of 3 mg/kg • Follow with a continuous infusion of 1 to 4 mg/min (reduced dose may be needed in the elderly and those with underlying liver disease) *If the drug has been given during cardiac arrest, start infusion as indicated. May give additional bolus for recurrent VF/VT up to 3 mg/kg; seek expert consultation.* **Note:** Prophylactic administration of lidocaine to patients with acute coronary syndromes is not recommended.

Pulseless Electrical Activity (PEA) Case

Introduction

This case focuses on assessment and management of a *cardiac arrest patient with pulseless electrical activity (PEA).* During the BLS Primary Survey, team members will demonstrate high-quality CPR with effective chest compressions and ventilation with a bag-mask. In the ACLS Secondary Survey, the team leader will recognize the rhythm of PEA and implement the appropriate interventions outlined in the Pulseless Arrest Algorithm. Because correction of an underlying cause of PEA, if present and identified, is critical to patient outcome, the team leader will verbalize the Differential Diagnosis while leading the resuscitation team in the search for and treatment of reversible causes.

Learning Objectives

At the end of this case you should be able to

1. Define and recognize PEA
2. Treat PEA according to the ACLS Pulseless Arrest Algorithm (Figure 9)
3. Recall the correct dosage and method of administering vasopressors (epinephrine and vasopressin) in PEA
4. Recall indications and correct dosage for atropine in PEA
5. Recall that the target of PEA treatment is the cause, not the rhythm
6. Recall the most likely causes of PEA
7. Assign team functions and monitor CPR

Rhythms for PEA

You will need to recognize the following rhythms:

- PEA
- Rate—too fast or too slow
- Width of QRS complexes—wide versus narrow

Drugs for PEA

This case involves these drugs:

- Epinephrine
- Vasopressin
- Atropine
- Other medications, depending on the cause of the PEA arrest

Description of PEA

Introduction

PEA encompasses a heterogeneous group of rhythms that are organized or semi-organized but lack a palpable pulse. PEA includes

- Idioventricular rhythms
- Ventricular escape rhythms
- Postdefibrillation idioventricular rhythms
- Bradyasystolic rhythms

Any organized rhythm without a pulse is defined as PEA. Even sinus rhythm without a detectable pulse is called PEA. Pulseless rhythms that are excluded by definition include VF, VT, and asystole.

Historical Perspective

Previously the term *electromechanical dissociation* (EMD) was used to describe patients who displayed electrical activity on the cardiac monitor but who lacked apparent contractile function because the pulse was not detectable. A more accurate and descriptive term to convey the meaning of this condition is *pulseless electrical activity*. In fact, most patients have a condition called pseudo-PEA. That is, weak contractile function is present—detectable by invasive monitoring or echocardiography—but the cardiac function is too weak to produce a pulse or effective cardiac output. This is the most common rhythm present following defibrillation.

Managing PEA: the ACLS Pulseless Arrest Algorithm

Overview

As described earlier, the ACLS Pulseless Arrest Algorithm consists of 2 pathways for a pulseless arrest (Figure 9). The pathway on the left side of the algorithm outlines the steps to take for a shockable rhythm (VF/VT). The pathway on the right side of the algorithm outlines the steps to take for a nonshockable rhythm (asystole/PEA). Because of the similarity in causes and management, the ACLS Pulseless Arrest Algorithm combines the asystole and PEA pathways. But we will review these rhythms in separate cases. In both pathways therapies are organized around periods (2 minutes or 5 cycles) of uninterrupted, high-quality CPR.

The ability to achieve a good resuscitation outcome, with return of a perfusing rhythm and spontaneous respirations, depends on the ability of the resuscitation team to provide effective CPR and to identify and correct a cause of PEA if present.

Everyone on the resuscitation team must carry out the steps outlined in the algorithm and, at the same time, focus on the search for and treatment of reversible causes of the arrest.

The PEA Pathway of the Pulseless Arrest Algorithm

In this case the *patient is in cardiac arrest.* Team members initiate and perform high-quality CPR throughout the BLS Primary Survey and the ACLS Secondary Survey. CPR is interrupted for ≤10 seconds for rhythm and pulse checks. *This patient has no pulse, and the rhythm on the monitor is PEA* (Box 9). Chest compressions resume immediately. The team leader now directs the team in the steps outlined in the PEA pathway of the Pulseless Arrest Algorithm (Figure 9), beginning with Box 10. IV/IO access is a priority over advanced airway management. All resuscitation team members must simultaneously conduct a search for an underlying and treatable cause of the PEA in addition to performing their assigned roles.

Administer Vasopressors (Box 10)

Continue high-quality CPR. As soon as IV/IO access is available, give a vasopressor:

- Epinephrine 1 mg IV/IO—repeat every 3 to 5 minutes

  OR

- Vasopressin 40 U IV/IO to replace first or second dose of epinephrine

---
Administer drugs during CPR. Do not stop CPR to administer drugs.

You can substitute a single dose of vasopressin 40 U IV/IO for either the first or second dose of epinephrine. But give vasopressin only once.

No vasopressor has been shown to increase survival from PEA. Because vasopressors (epinephrine and vasopressin) can improve aortic diastolic blood pressure and coronary artery perfusion pressure, they continue to be recommended. The efficacy of vasopressin does not differ substantially from that of epinephrine; it is included as an option.

Consider Atropine (Box 10)

If the PEA rate is *slow,* consider giving atropine as follows:

- Atropine 1 mg IV/IO—repeat every 3 to 5 minutes (up to 3 doses)

A shorter dosing interval (every 3 minutes) for atropine is possibly helpful in cardiac arrest.

Rhythm Check: Decision Point (Box 11)

Box 11 directs you to give 2 minutes (about 5 cycles) of CPR after administration of the drugs and then conduct a rhythm check. Be careful to minimize interruptions in chest compressions.

The pause in CPR to conduct a rhythm check should not exceed 10 seconds.

Nonshockable Rhythm (Box 12)

If *no electrical activity is present* (asystole), go back to Box 10.

If organized electrical activity is present, try to palpate a pulse. Take at least 5 seconds but do not take more than 10 seconds to check for a pulse.

If *no pulse is present*, or if there is any doubt about the presence of a pulse, immediately resume CPR, starting with chest compressions. Go back to Box 10 and repeat the sequence.

If a palpable pulse is present and the rhythm is organized, begin post-resuscitative care.

Decision Point: Shockable (Box 13)

If the rhythm check reveals a shockable rhythm, resume CPR with chest compressions while the defibrillator is charging if possible. You now switch to the left side of the algorithm and perform steps according to the VF/VT sequence starting with Box 4.

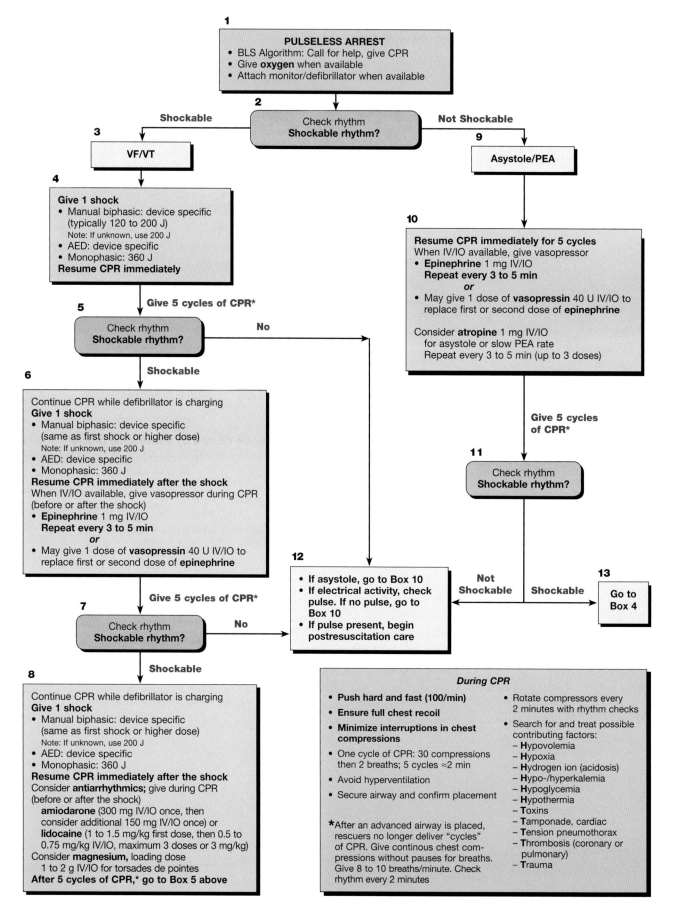

1

PULSELESS ARREST
• BLS Algorithm: Call for help, give CPR
• Give **oxygen** when available
• Attach monitor/defibrillator when available

2

Check rhythm
Shockable rhythm?

Shockable ← | → Not Shockable

3

VF/VT

9

Asystole/PEA

4

Give 1 shock
• Manual biphasic: device specific
  (typically 120 to 200 J)
  Note: If unknown, use 200 J
• AED: device specific
• Monophasic: 360 J
Resume CPR immediately

Give 5 cycles of CPR*

5

Check rhythm
Shockable rhythm?

No →

Shockable ↓

6

Continue CPR while defibrillator is charging
Give 1 shock
• Manual biphasic: device specific
  (same as first shock or higher dose)
  Note: If unknown, use 200 J
• AED: device specific
• Monophasic: 360 J
Resume CPR immediately after the shock
When IV/IO available, give vasopressor during CPR
(before or after the shock)
• **Epinephrine** 1 mg IV/IO
  Repeat every 3 to 5 min
      or
• May give 1 dose of **vasopressin** 40 U IV/IO to
  replace first or second dose of **epinephrine**

Give 5 cycles of CPR*

7

Check rhythm
Shockable rhythm?

No →

Shockable ↓

8

Continue CPR while defibrillator is charging
Give 1 shock
• Manual biphasic: device specific
  (same as first shock or higher dose)
  Note: If unknown, use 200 J
• AED: device specific
• Monophasic: 360 J
Resume CPR immediately after the shock
Consider **antiarrhythmics;** give during CPR
(before or after the shock)
  amiodarone (300 mg IV/IO once, then
  consider additional 150 mg IV/IO once) or
  lidocaine (1 to 1.5 mg/kg first dose, then 0.5 to
  0.75 mg/kg IV/IO, maximum 3 doses or 3 mg/kg)
Consider **magnesium,** loading dose
  1 to 2 g IV/IO for torsades de pointes
After 5 cycles of CPR,* go to Box 5 above

10

Resume CPR immediately for 5 cycles
When IV/IO available, give vasopressor
• **Epinephrine** 1 mg IV/IO
  Repeat every 3 to 5 min
      or
• May give 1 dose of **vasopressin** 40 U IV/IO to
  replace first or second dose of **epinephrine**

Consider **atropine** 1 mg IV/IO
  for asystole or slow PEA rate
  Repeat every 3 to 5 min (up to 3 doses)

Give 5 cycles
of CPR*

11

Check rhythm
Shockable rhythm?

Not Shockable | Shockable

12

• If asystole, go to Box 10
• If electrical activity, check
  pulse. If no pulse, go to
  Box 10
• If pulse present, begin
  postresuscitation care

13

Go to
Box 4

During CPR

• **Push hard and fast (100/min)**
• **Ensure full chest recoil**
• **Minimize interruptions in chest
  compressions**
• One cycle of CPR: 30 compressions
  then 2 breaths; 5 cycles ≈2 min
• Avoid hyperventilation
• Secure airway and confirm placement

*After an advanced airway is placed,
rescuers no longer deliver "cycles"
of CPR. Give continous chest compressions without pauses for breaths.
Give 8 to 10 breaths/minute. Check
rhythm every 2 minutes

• Rotate compressors every
  2 minutes with rhythm checks
• Search for and treat possible
  contributing factors:
  – **H**ypovolemia
  – **H**ypoxia
  – **H**ydrogen ion (acidosis)
  – **H**ypo-/hyperkalemia
  – **H**ypoglycemia
  – **H**ypothermia
  – **T**oxins
  – **T**amponade, cardiac
  – **T**ension pneumothorax
  – **T**hrombosis (coronary or
    pulmonary)
  – **T**rauma

Figure 9. ACLS Pulseless Arrest Algorithm.

Asystole and PEA Treatment Sequences

The diagram in Figure 10 summarizes the recommended sequence of CPR, rhythm checks, and delivery of drugs for PEA and asystole based on expert consensus.

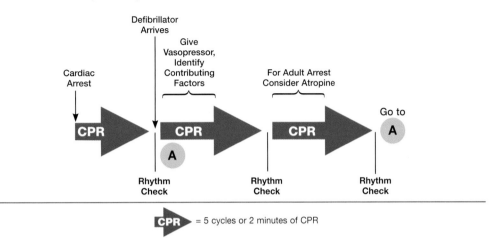

Figure 10. Pulseless Arrest: Treatment Sequences–Asystole/PEA. Prepare next drug prior to rhythm check. Administer drug during CPR, as soon as possible after the rhythm check confirms no VF/pulseless VT. Continue CPR while drugs are prepared and administered. Ideally, chest compressions should be interrupted only for ventilation (until advanced airway placed) and rhythm check. Search for and treat possible contributing factors.

Managing PEA: Diagnosing and Treating Underlying Causes

Introduction

Patients with PEA have poor outcomes. Rapid assessment and aggressive management offer the best chance of success. PEA may be caused by a reversible problem. If you can quickly identify a specific condition that has caused or is contributing to PEA and correct it, you may achieve ROSC. The identification of the underlying cause is of paramount importance in cases of PEA and asystole.

In the search for the underlying cause, do the following:

- Consider frequent causes of PEA by recalling the H's and T's
- Analyze the ECG for clues to the underlying cause
- Recognize hypovolemia
- Recognize drug overdose/poisonings

H's and T's

PEA is associated with many conditions. If you don't think about a possible cause, you might not recognize it. Memorize the following list of common causes to keep from overlooking an obvious cause of PEA that might be reversed by appropriate treatment.

The most common causes of PEA are presented as H's and T's in the table below:

H's	T's
Hypovolemia	**T**oxins
Hypoxia	**T**amponade (cardiac)
Hydrogen ion (acidosis)	**T**ension pneumothorax
Hyper-/hypokalemia	**T**hrombosis (coronary and pulmonary)
Hypoglycemia	**T**rauma
Hypothermia	

Conditions and Management

The factors in the patient's history and physical exam that may help identify reversible causes of PEA have been combined with recommendations for management in Table 3.

Table 3. Frequent Causes of PEA (H's and T's)

Condition	Clues From ECG and Monitor	Clues From History and Physical Exam	Recommended Treatment
Hypo-volemia	Narrow complex Rapid rate	History, flat neck veins	Volume infusion
Hypoxia	Slow rate (hypoxia)	Cyanosis, blood gases, airway problems	Oxygenation, ventilation
Hydrogen ion (acidosis)	Smaller-amplitude QRS complexes	History of diabetes, bicarbonate-responsive preexisting acidosis, renal failure	Sodium bicarbonate, hyperventilation
Hyper-kalemia or	Both hyperkalemia and hypokalemia cause wide-complex QRS *"High potassium" ECG:* • T waves taller and peaked • P waves get smaller • QRS widens • Sine-wave PEA	History of renal failure, diabetes, recent dialysis, dialysis fistulas, medications	*Hyperkalemia:* • Sodium bicarbonate • Glucose plus insulin • Calcium chloride • Kayexalate/ sorbitol • Dialysis (long term) • Possibly albuterol
Hypo-kalemia	*"Low potassium" ECG:* • T waves flatten • Prominent U waves • QRS widens • QT prolongs • Wide-complex tachycardia	Abnormal loss of potassium, diuretic use	*Hypokalemia:* • Rapid but controlled infusion of potassium • Add magnesium if cardiac arrest
Hypo-thermia	J or Osborne waves	History of exposure to cold, central body temperature	See Hypothermia Algorithm (ECC Handbook)

Condition	Clues From ECG and Monitor	Clues From History and Physical Exam	Recommended Treatment
Tablets (drug overdose): tricyclics, digoxin, β-blockers, calcium channel blockers	Various effects on ECG, predominately prolongation of QT interval	Bradycardia, empty bottles at the scene, pupils, neurologic exam	Drug screens, intubation, lavage, activated charcoal, lactulose per local protocols, specific antidotes and agents per toxidrome
Tamponade, cardiac	Narrow complex Rapid rate	History, no pulse felt with CPR, vein distention	Pericardiocentesis
Tension pneumothorax	Narrow complex Slow rate (hypoxia)	History, no pulse felt with CPR, neck vein distention, tracheal deviation, unequal breath sounds, difficult to ventilate patient	Needle decompression
Thrombosis, heart: acute, massive MI	Abnormal 12-lead ECG: • Q waves • ST-segment changes • T waves, inversions	History, cardiac markers	Fibrinolytic agents; see the STEMI Case
Thrombosis, lungs: massive pulmonary embolism	Narrow complex Rapid rate	History, no pulse felt with CPR, distended neck veins, prior positive test for DVT or PE	Surgical embolectomy, fibrinolytics

Analyze ECG for Clues to Underlying Cause

The ECG may provide valuable clues to the possible causes of PEA. Many providers think that the term *PEA* refers to the broad, slurred, slow, and disorganized electrical activity that bears no similarity to a normal P wave-QRS-T wave complex. The ECG, however, may display normal intervals or complexes or both. For example, sinus rhythm due to hypovolemia or sepsis may present as PEA. Other ECG findings in PEA may include wide-complex QRS.

Reassess the monitored rhythm and note the rate and width of the QRS complexes (Table 4). Without interrupting CPR for more than about 10 seconds, obtain a 12-lead ECG if possible. Newer ECG machines can record a 12-lead in a few seconds.

Table 4. Classification of PEA Rhythms by Rate and QRS Width

Rate of Complexes	Width of Complexes	
	Narrow More likely to have noncardiac cause; low volume, low vascular tone	*Wide* More often due to cardiac cause; also drug and electrolyte toxicities
Fast (>60 bpm)	• Sinus (P wave) PEA • Pseudo-PEA • Reentry SVT	• VF • VT
Slow (<60 bpm)	• PEA • Pseudo-PEA • Postdefibrillation • Idioventricular rhythms	• Bradyasystolic rhythms • Idioventricular rhythms • Ventricular escape rhythms

Hypovolemia

Hypovolemia, a common cause of PEA, initially produces the classic physiologic response of a *rapid, narrow-complex tachycardia (sinus tachycardia)* and typically produces increased diastolic and decreased systolic pressures. As loss of blood volume continues, blood pressure drops, eventually becoming undetectable, but the narrow QRS complexes and rapid rate continue (ie, PEA).

You should consider hypovolemia as a cause of hypotension, which can deteriorate to PEA. Providing prompt treatment can then reverse the pulseless state by rapidly correcting the hypovolemia. Common nontraumatic causes of hypovolemia include occult internal hemorrhage and severe dehydration. Consider volume infusion for PEA associated with a narrow-complex tachycardia.

Cardiac and Pulmonary Conditions

Acute coronary ischemia involving a large amount of heart muscle can present as PEA. That is, occlusion of the left main or proximal left anterior descending coronary artery can present with cardiogenic shock rapidly progressing to cardiac arrest and PEA. Massive or saddle pulmonary embolism obstructs flow to the pulmonary vasculature and causes acute right heart failure. Although there have been case reports of successful resuscitation following administration of fibrinolytic therapy, one large clinical trial of in-hospital and out-of-hospital cardiac arrest failed to show benefit.

Cardiac tamponade may be a reversible condition. Volume infusion in this condition may also help while definitive therapy is initiated. Tension pneumothorax can be effectively treated once recognized.

Note that cardiac tamponade, tension pneumothorax, and massive pulmonary embolism cannot be treated unless recognized. Bedside ultrasound, when performed by a skilled provider, may aid in rapid identification of tamponade and pulmonary embolism. There is growing evidence that pneumothorax can be identified using bedside ultrasound as well. Treatment for cardiac tamponade may require pericardiocentesis. Tension pneumothorax requires needle aspiration and chest tube placement. These procedures are beyond the scope of the ACLS Provider Course.

Drug Overdoses or Toxic Exposures

Certain drug overdoses and toxic exposures may lead to peripheral vascular dilatation and/or myocardial dysfunction with resultant hypotension. These are another cause of PEA. The approach to poisoned patients should be aggressive because the toxic effects may progress rapidly and may be of limited duration. In these situations myocardial dysfunction and arrhythmias may be reversible. Numerous case reports confirm the success of many specific limited interventions with one thing in common—they buy time.

Treatments are designed to support a viable level of blood flow to the brain, heart, and other vital organs while awaiting correction of specific electrolyte abnormalities or toxic blood levels of drugs or poisons. Treatments that can provide this level of support include

- Prolonged basic CPR in special resuscitation situations
- Cardiopulmonary bypass
- Intra-aortic balloon pumping
- Renal dialysis
- Specific drug antidotes (digibind, glucagon, bicarbonate)
- Transcutaneous pacing
- Correction of severe electrolyte disturbances (potassium, magnesium, calcium, acidosis)
- Specific adjunctive agents (eg, naloxone)

Critical Concepts:

Common Reversible Causes of PEA

Hypovolemia and hypoxia are the two most common and easily reversible causes of PEA. Be sure to look for evidence of these problems as you assess the patient.

Asystole Case

Introduction

In this case the *patient is in cardiac arrest.* Team members initiate and perform high-quality CPR throughout the BLS Primary Survey and the ACLS Secondary Survey. CPR is interrupted for ≤10 seconds for rhythm and pulse checks. *This patient has no pulse, and the rhythm on the monitor is Asystole.* Chest compressions resume immediately. The team leader now directs the team in the steps outlined in the Asystole pathway of the Pulseless Arrest Algorithm (Figure 9 on page 54), beginning with Box 10. IV/IO access is a priority over advanced airway management. All resuscitation team members must simultaneously conduct a search for an underlying and treatable cause of the PEA in addition to performing their assigned roles. At the end of this case the team will discuss the criteria for terminating resuscitative efforts; in some cases we must recognize that the patient is dead and that it would be more appropriate to direct efforts to supporting the family.

Learning Objectives	At the end of the case you should be able to
	1. Discuss the circumstances when resuscitation should not be initiated
	2. Recall that survival from asystole is poor and that asystole may represent an agonal end-stage rhythm
	3. Recall that asystole and PEA are treated similarly, may have like causes, and require an early diligent search for a reversible cause
	4. Recognize a do-not-attempt-resuscitation (DNAR) order
	5. Recall the reversible causes of asystole and outline the treatment of each
	6. Follow the ACLS Pulseless Arrest Algorithm as it applies to asystole
	7. Recall the correct dosage and timing of administration for epinephrine, vasopressin, and atropine in cardiac arrest
	8. Assign team member roles and monitor performance

Rhythms for Asystole

You will need to recognize the following rhythms:

- Asystole
- Slow PEA terminating in bradyasystolic rhythm

Drugs for Asystole

This case involves these drugs:

- Atropine
- Epinephrine
- Vasopressin

Approach to Asystole

Introduction

Asystole is a cardiac arrest rhythm associated with no discernible electrical activity on the ECG (also referred to as *flat line*). You should confirm that the flat line on the monitor is indeed "true asystole" by validating that the flat line is

- Not another rhythm (eg, fine VF) masquerading as a flat line
- Not the result of an operator error that is creating a flat line (ie, asystole) on the monitor when in reality another rhythm is present

---

Foundation Facts:

Asystole and Technical Problems

Asystole is a specific diagnosis, but flat line is not. The term *flat line* is nonspecific and could result from several possible conditions, including absence of cardiac electrical activity, lead or other equipment failure, and operator error. Some defibrillators and monitors signal the operator when a lead or other equipment failure occurs. Some of these problems are not applicable to all defibrillators.

For a patient with pulseless arrest and asystole, quickly rule out any other causes of an isoelectric ECG, such as

- Loose leads or leads not connected to the patient or defibrillator/monitor
- No power
- Signal gain (amplitude/signal strength) too low

Patients With DNAR Orders

During the BLS Primary Survey and ACLS Secondary Survey, you should be aware of reasons to stop or withhold resuscitative efforts. Some of these are

- Rigor mortis
- Indicators of DNAR status (eg, bracelet, anklet, written documentation)
- Family or personal information (living will)
- Threat to safety of rescuers

Out-of-hospital providers need to be aware of EMS-specific policies and protocols applicable to these situations. In-hospital providers and resuscitation teams should be aware of advance directives or specific limits to resuscitation attempts that are in place. That is, some patients may consent to CPR and defibrillation but not to intubation or invasive procedures. Many hospitals will record this in the medical record.

Asystole as an End Point

The prognosis for cardiac arrest with asystole is very poor. A large percentage of asystolic patients do not survive. In hospital, asystole occurs mostly in severely ill patients, and it is often the end point of a prolonged illness or cardiac arrest. Often asystole represents the final rhythm of a patient whose organs have failed and whose condition has deteriorated. Cardiac function has diminished until electrical and functional cardiac activity finally stop and the patient dies. Asystole is also the final rhythm of a patient initially in VF or VT.

In such scenarios attempted resuscitation may not be appropriate. Prolonged efforts are unnecessary and futile unless special resuscitation situations exist, such as hypothermia and drug overdose.

Managing Asystole

Overview

The management of asystole consists of the following components:

- Implementing the steps in the Pulseless Arrest Algorithm
- Identification and correction of underlying causes
- Terminating efforts as appropriate

Pulseless Arrest Algorithm

As described in the VF/pulseless VT and PEA cases, the ACLS Pulseless Arrest Algorithm consists of 2 pathways for a pulseless arrest (Figure 9, previous case). The pathway on the left side of the algorithm outlines the steps to take for a shockable rhythm (VF/pulseless VT). The pathway on the right side of the algorithm outlines the steps to take for a nonshockable rhythm (asystole/PEA). In both pathways therapies are designed around periods (5 cycles or 2 minutes) of uninterrupted, high-quality CPR. In this case we will focus on the asystole component of the asystole/PEA pathway.

Identification and Correction of Underlying Cause

Treatment of asystole is not limited to the interventions outlined in the algorithm. Efforts should be made to identify and correct an underlying cause if present. Rescuers must stop, think, and ask, "Why did *this* person have *this* cardiac arrest at *this* time?" It is essential to search for and treat reversible causes of asystole for resuscitative efforts to be potentially successful. Use the H's and T's to recall conditions that could have contributed to asystole:

H's	T's
Hypovolemia	**T**oxins
Hypoxia	**T**amponade (cardiac)
Hydrogen ion (acidosis)	**T**ension pneumothorax
Hyper-/hypokalemia	**T**hrombosis (coronary and pulmonary)
Hypoglycemia	**T**rauma
Hypothermia	

See the PEA case for more information on the H's and T's, including clinical clues and suggested treatments.

Application of the Pulseless Arrest Algorithm—Asystole Pathway

Introduction

In this case you have a patient in cardiac arrest. High-quality CPR is performed throughout the BLS Primary Survey and the ACLS Secondary Survey. Interrupt CPR for ≤10 seconds while you perform a rhythm and pulse check. This patient has no pulse. You interpret the rhythm on the monitor as asystole. CPR beginning with chest compressions resumes immediately. You now conduct the steps outlined in the *asystole pathway of the Pulseless Arrest Algorithm* beginning with Box 9. At the same time you are searching for a possible underlying cause of the asystole.

Confirmed Asystole (Box 9)

Give priority to IV/IO access. Do not routinely insert an advanced airway unless ventilations with a bag-mask are ineffective. Do not interrupt CPR while establishing IV or IO access.

Administer Vasopressors (Box 10)

Continue high-quality CPR, and as soon as IV/IO access is available, give a vasopressor as follows:

- **Epinephrine** 1 mg IV/IO—repeat every 3 to 5 minutes
  OR
- **Vasopressin** 40 U IV/IO to replace the first or second dose of epinephrine

> *Administer drugs during CPR. Do not stop CPR to administer drugs.*

You can substitute vasopressin for either the first or second dose of epinephrine. But it can be given only once. In a large study of vasopressin versus epinephrine for cardiac arrest, a post-hoc analysis of the subgroup of patients with asystole showed improved survival following administration of vasopressin but no improvement in neurologic outcome.

Consider Atropine (Box 10)

Atropine sulfate reverses cholinergic-mediated decreases in heart rate, systemic vascular resistance, and blood pressure. No prospective controlled studies support its use in asystole. A retrospective review of intubated patients with refractory asystole showed improved rates of survival to hospital admission with atropine.

Asystole can be exacerbated or precipitated by excessive vagal tone, so it is logical to consider using a drug with vagolytic effects. For asystole, consider

- Atropine 1 mg IV/IO—repeat every 3 to 5 minutes (up to 3 doses)

Decision Point: Rhythm Check (Box 11)

Box 11 directs you to check the rhythm after 2 minutes (about 5 cycles) of CPR. Be careful to minimize interruptions in chest compressions.

> *Interruption of chest compressions to conduct a rhythm or pulse check should not exceed 10 seconds.*

Nonshockable (Box 12)

If *no electrical activity is present* (asystole), go back to Box 10.

If electrical activity is present, try to palpate a pulse.

If *no pulse is present* or if there is any doubt about the presence of a pulse, continue CPR, starting with chest compressions. Go back to Box 10 and repeat the sequence.

If a *good pulse is present and the rhythm is organized,* begin postresuscitative care.

Shockable (Box 13)

If the rhythm check reveals a shockable rhythm, you will prepare to deliver a shock (resuming chest compressions during charging if appropriate). You will now refer to the left side of the algorithm and perform steps according to the VF/VT sequence starting with Box 4.

Asystole and PEA Treatment Sequences

The diagram in Figure 10 (in previous case, PEA) summarizes the recommended sequence of CPR, rhythm checks, and delivery of drugs for PEA and asystole based on expert consensus.

Transcutaneous Pacing Not Recommended

Several randomized controlled trials failed to show benefit from attempted transcutaneous pacing (TCP) for asystole. At this time the use of pacing for patients with asystolic cardiac arrest is not recommended.

Routine Shock Administration Not Recommended

There is no evidence that attempting to "defibrillate" asystole is beneficial. In one study the group that received shocks had a trend toward worse outcome. Given the importance of minimizing interruption of chest compressions, there is no justification for interrupting chest compressions to deliver a shock to patients with asystole.

When in Doubt

If it is unclear whether the rhythm is fine VF or asystole, an initial attempt at defibrillation may be warranted. Fine VF may be the result of a prolonged arrest. Before defibrillation, rescuers may consider a period (2 minutes or about 5 cycles) of high-quality CPR.

Terminating Resuscitative Efforts

Terminating In-Hospital Resuscitative Efforts

If a reversible cause is not rapidly identified and the patient fails to respond to the BLS Primary Survey and ACLS Secondary Survey management, termination of resuscitative efforts may be appropriate.

The decision to terminate resuscitative efforts rests with the treating physician in the hospital and is based on consideration of many factors, including

- Time to CPR
- Time to defibrillation
- Comorbid disease
- Prearrest state
- Initial arrest rhythm
- Response to resuscitative measures

None of these factors alone or in combination is clearly predictive of outcome. The duration of resuscitative efforts, however, is an important factor associated with poor outcome. The chance that the patient will be discharged from the hospital alive and neurologically intact diminishes as resuscitation time increases. Stop the resuscitation attempt when you determine with a high degree of certainty that the patient will not respond to further ACLS.

Terminating Out-of-Hospital Resuscitative Efforts

Continue out-of-hospital resuscitative efforts until one of the following occurs:

- Restoration of effective, spontaneous circulation and ventilation
- Transfer of care to a senior emergency medical professional who may determine that the patient is unresponsive to resuscitation
- The presence of reliable criteria indicating irreversible death
- The rescuer is unable to continue because of exhaustion or dangerous environmental hazards or because continued resuscitation places the lives of others in jeopardy
- A valid DNAR order is presented
- Online authorization from the medical control physician or by prior medical protocol for termination of resuscitation

Duration of Resuscitative Efforts

Available scientific studies have shown that in the absence of mitigating factors, prolonged resuscitative efforts are unlikely to be successful and that they can be discontinued if there is no ROSC at any time during, or following, 20 minutes of cumulative BLS and ACLS. If ROSC of any duration occurs, it may be appropriate to consider extending the resuscitative effort. Clinical rules have been developed to assist in decisions to terminate resuscitative efforts for in-hospital and out-of-hospital arrests. You should familiarize yourself with established policy or protocols for your hospital or EMS system.

It may also be appropriate to consider other issues, such as drug overdose and severe prearrest hypothermia (eg, submersion in icy water) when deciding whether to extend resuscitative efforts. Special resuscitation interventions and prolonged resuscitative efforts may be indicated for patients with hypothermia, drug overdose, or other potentially reversible causes of arrest.

Asystole—An Agonal Rhythm Confirming Death

You will see asystole most frequently in 2 situations:

- As a terminal rhythm in a resuscitation attempt that started with another rhythm
- As the first rhythm identified in a patient with unwitnessed or prolonged arrest

In either of these scenarios, asystole most often represents an agonal rhythm confirming death rather than a "rhythm" to be treated or a patient who can be resuscitated if the attempt persists long enough. Persistent asystole represents extensive myocardial ischemia and damage from prolonged periods of inadequate coronary perfusion. Prognosis is very poor unless a special resuscitation circumstance or immediately reversible cause is present. Survival from asystole is better for in-hospital than for out-of-hospital arrests according to data from the National Registry of CPR (www.nrcpr.org).

Ethical Considerations

The resuscitation team must make a conscientious and competent effort to give patients "a trial of CPR and ACLS" provided the patient had not expressed a decision to forego resuscitative efforts (see the DNAR discussion on the student CD). The final decision to stop resuscitative efforts can never be as simple as an isolated time interval.

See Human, Ethical, and Legal Dimensions of CPR on the student CD.

Transport of Patients in Cardiac Arrest

Emergency medical response systems should not require field personnel to transport every victim of cardiac arrest back to a hospital or to an emergency department (ED). Transportation with continuing CPR is justified if interventions available in the ED cannot be performed in the out-of-hospital setting and they are indicated for special circumstances (ie, cardiopulmonary bypass or extracorporeal circulation for patients of severe hypothermia).

Acute Coronary Syndromes Case

Introduction

The ACLS provider must have the basic knowledge to assess and stabilize patients with acute coronary syndromes (ACS). *Patients in this case have signs and symptoms of ACS, including possible acute myocardial infarction (AMI).* You will use the Acute Coronary Syndromes Algorithm as the guide to clinical strategy.

The initial 12-lead ECG is used in all ACS cases to classify patients into 1 of 3 ECG categories, each with different assessment and management needs. These 3 ECG categories are ST-segment elevation, ST-segment depression, and nondiagnostic or normal ECG. These are outlined in the Acute Coronary Syndrome Algorithm (Figure 12) and they are covered in ACLS courses as follows:

- The **ACLS Provider Course** emphasizes the *ST-segment elevation myocardial infarction (STEMI)* treatment arm and early identification of STEMI patients for rapid reperfusion. Although providers do not need to possess the skills to interpret a 12-lead ECG, the ability to recognize ST-segment elevation suspicious for STEMI and triage for prompt reperfusion therapy are goals of this case.

- The **ACLS Experienced Provider Course** includes assessment, triage, and treatment for high-risk *unstable angina and non–ST-elevation myocardial infarction (NSTEMI)* patients (middle treatment arm of the algorithm) and *low-risk or nonspecific chest pain* patients (right treatment arm of the algorithm). Experienced providers may have 12-lead ECG interpretation skills. The ACLS Experienced Provider Course includes further discussion of patients with the spectrum of ACS.

Key components of this case are

- Identification and treatment of acute ischemic chest pain
- Initial treatment of possible acute ischemic syndromes
- Emphasis on early reperfusion of the patient with STEMI

Learning Objectives

At the end of this case you should be able to

1. Discuss the differential diagnosis of life-threatening chest discomfort
2. Explain and apply the ACLS ACS Algorithm (Figure 12), including the initial use of drugs, doses, and strategies
3. Understand and explain early identification, risk stratification, and treatment of patients with ACS
4. Explain actions, indications, precautions, contraindications, dosage, and administration for oxygen, aspirin, nitroglycerin, morphine, fibrinolytic therapy, and heparin (low-molecular-weight heparin [LMWH] or unfractionated heparin [UFH]) in patients with possible ACS
5. Understand and be able to explain guidelines for reperfusion strategies

Rhythms for ACS

Sudden cardiac death due to VF and bradycardic hypotensive rhythms occurs with acute ischemia. Providers will understand to anticipate these rhythms and be prepared for immediate attempts at defibrillation and administration of drug or electrical therapy for symptomatic bradyarrhythmias.

Although 12-lead ECG interpretation is beyond the scope of the basic ACLS Provider Course, some ACLS providers will have 12-lead ECG reading skills. For them this case summarizes the identification and management of patients with STEMI.

Drugs for ACS

Drug therapy and treatment strategies continue to evolve rapidly in the field of ACS. ACLS providers and instructors will need to monitor important changes. Only basic knowledge is presented in the ACLS Provider Course with the intent to focus early treatment on the priority of rapid reperfusion, relief of ischemic pain, and treatment of early life-threatening complications. Reperfusion may involve the use of fibrinolytic therapy or percutaneous coronary intervention (PCI, ie, balloon angioplasty/stent).

Treatment of ACS involves the initial use of drugs to relieve ischemic discomfort, dissolve clots, and inhibit thrombin and platelets. These drugs are

- Oxygen
- Aspirin
- Nitroglycerin
- Morphine
- Fibrinolytic therapy (overview)
- Heparin (unfractionated [UFH], low molecular weight [LWMH])

Additional agents that are adjunctive to initial therapy and will not be discussed in the ACLS Provider Course are

- β-Blockers
- Clopidogrel
- Angiotensin-converting enzyme (ACE) inhibitors
- HMG-CoA reductase inhibitor (statin therapy)

Goals for ACS Patients

Foundation Facts:

Out-of-Hospital Cardiac Arrest Response

Half of the patients who die of ACS do so before reaching the hospital. VF or pulseless VT is the precipitating rhythm in most of these deaths. VF is most likely to develop during the first 4 hours after onset of symptoms.

Communities should develop programs to respond to out-of-hospital cardiac arrest. Such programs should focus on

- Recognizing symptoms of ACS
- Activating the EMS system with EMS advance notification of the receiving hospital
- Providing early CPR
- Providing early defibrillation with AEDs available through public access defibrillation programs and first responders
- Providing a coordinated system of care among the EMS system, the ED, and Cardiology

Goals of Therapy

The primary goal of therapy for patients with ACS is identification of patients with STEMI and triage for early reperfusion therapy.

Reperfusion therapy opens an occluded coronary artery with either drugs or mechanical means. "Clot buster" drugs are called *fibrinolytics*—a more accurate term than *thrombolytics*. PCI, performed in the heart catheterization suite following coronary angiography, allows balloon dilation and/or stent placement for an occluded coronary artery. PCI performed as the initial reperfusion method is called *primary* PCI.

Other, secondary important goals are

- Relief of ischemic chest discomfort
- Prevention of major adverse cardiac events (MACE), such as death, nonfatal MI, and the need for post-infarction urgent revascularization
- Treatment of acute, life-threatening complications of ACS, such as VF/pulseless VT, symptomatic bradycardias, and unstable tachycardias

Pathophysiology of ACS

Acute coronary syndromes (Figure 11). Patients with coronary atherosclerosis may develop a spectrum of clinical syndromes representing varying degrees of coronary artery occlusion. These syndromes include unstable angina (UA), non–ST-segment elevation MI (NSTEMI) and ST-segment elevation MI (STEMI). Sudden cardiac death may occur with each of these syndromes.

A Unstable plaque. Rupture of a lipid-laden plaque with a thin cap is the most common cause of an ACS. The majority of these plaques are not hemodynamically significant before rupture. An inflammatory component is present in the subendothelial area and further weakens and predisposes the plaque to rupture. Blood flow velocity, turbulence, and vessel anatomy may be important contributing factors. Superficial erosion of a plaque occurs in a small percentage of patients.

B Plaque rupture. After rupture a monolayer of platelets covers the surface of the ruptured plaque (platelet adhesion). Additional platelets are recruited (platelet aggregation) and activated. Fibrinogen cross-links platelets, and the coagulation system is activated with thrombin generation.

C Unstable angina. A partially occluding thrombus produces symptoms of ischemia, which are prolonged and may occur at rest. At this stage the thrombus is platelet-rich. Therapy with antiplatelet agents such as aspirin, clopidogrel, and glycoprotein IIb/IIIa receptor inhibitors is most effective at this time. Fibrinolytic therapy is not effective and may paradoxically accelerate occlusion by the release of clot-bound thrombin, which further activates platelets. An intermittently occlusive thrombus may cause myocardial necrosis, producing NSTEMI.

D Microemboli. As the clot enlarges, microemboli may originate from the distal thrombus and lodge in the coronary microvasculature, causing small elevations of cardiac troponins, sensitive cardiac markers for necrosis. These patients are at highest risk for progression to STEMI.

E Occlusive thrombus. If the thrombus completely occludes the coronary vessel for a prolonged period, STEMI occurs. This clot is rich in thrombin; early/prompt fibrinolysis or primary PCI may limit infarct size if performed sufficiently early.

Figure 11. Pathophysiology of acute coronary syndromes.

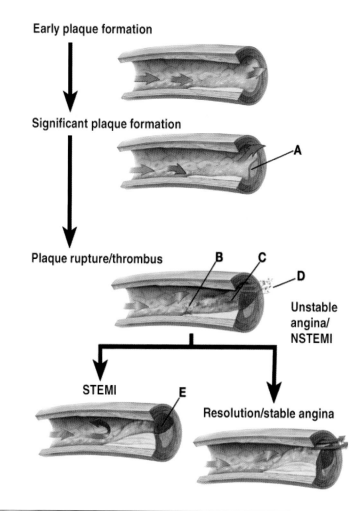

Early plaque formation

Significant plaque formation

A

Plaque rupture/thrombus

B C

D

Unstable angina/ NSTEMI

STEMI

E

Resolution/stable angina

Managing ACS: the Acute Coronary Syndromes Algorithm

Overview of the Algorithm

The Acute Coronary Syndromes Algorithm (Figure 12) outlines the steps for assessment and management of a patient presenting with ACS. Implementation of this algorithm begins with the identification of chest discomfort suggestive of ischemia (Box 1). The EMS responder in the out-of-hospital environment can begin immediate assessments and actions. These include giving oxygen, aspirin, nitroglycerin, and possibly morphine and obtaining an initial 12-lead ECG. Based on the ECG findings, the EMS provider may complete a fibrinolytic therapy checklist and notify the receiving ED of a potential AMI-STEMI when appropriate. If these initial steps were not initiated or completed before the patient's arrival at the hospital, the ED provider implements this component of care.

Subsequent treatment occurs upon arrival at the hospital. The out-of-hospital 12-lead ECG is reviewed if available. If one is not available, the emergency physician obtains it. The goal is to analyze the 12-lead ECG within 10 minutes of patient arrival at the ED. Patients are classified into 3 groups according to the analysis of the ST-segment on the 12-lead ECG. Treatment options are then recommended according to each group as follows:

- ST-Elevation MI (STEMI)
- High-Risk Unstable Angina (UA)/Non–ST-Elevation MI (NSTEMI)
- Intermediate/Low-Risk Unstable Angina (UA)

The Acute Coronary Syndromes Case will focus on the early reperfusion of the STEMI patient, emphasizing initial care and rapid triage for reperfusion therapy.

Important Considerations

The Acute Coronary Syndromes Algorithm (Figure 12) provides general guidelines that apply to the initial triage of patients based on symptoms and the 12-lead ECG. Serial cardiac markers (CK-MB, cardiac troponins) are obtained in most patients and allow additional risk stratification and treatment recommendations. Two important points for STEMI need emphasis:

- The ECG is central to the initial risk and treatment stratification.
- Reports of elevated cardiac markers are not necessary for a decision to administer fibrinolytic therapy or perform coronary intervention (angioplasty/stent).

Application of the ACS Algorithm

The boxes in the algorithm guide assessment and treatment as follows:

- Identification of chest discomfort suggestive of ischemia (Box 1)
- EMS assessment, care, transport, and hospital prearrival notification (Box 2)
- Immediate ED assessment and treatment (Box 3)
- Classification of patients according to the ST-segment analysis (Boxes 5, 9, 13)
- STEMI (Boxes 5 through 8)

Identification of Chest Discomfort Suggestive of Ischemia (Box 1)

Signs and Conditions

You should know how to identify chest discomfort suggestive of ischemia. Conduct a prompt and targeted evaluation of every patient whose initial complaints might suggest possible ACS.

The most common symptom of myocardial ischemia and infarction is retrosternal chest discomfort. The patient may perceive this discomfort more as pressure or tightness than actual pain.

Symptoms suggestive of ACS may also include

- Uncomfortable pressure, fullness, squeezing, or pain in the center of the chest lasting several minutes (usually more than a few minutes)
- Chest discomfort spreading to the shoulders, neck, one or both arms, or jaw
- Chest discomfort spreading into the back or between the shoulder blades
- Chest discomfort with lightheadedness, fainting, sweating, or nausea
- Unexplained, sudden shortness of breath, which may occur with or without chest discomfort

Consider the likelihood that the presenting condition is ACS or one of its potentially lethal mimics. Other life-threatening conditions besides ACS that may cause acute chest pain or discomfort are aortic dissection, acute pulmonary embolism, acute pericardial effusion with tamponade, and tension pneumothorax.

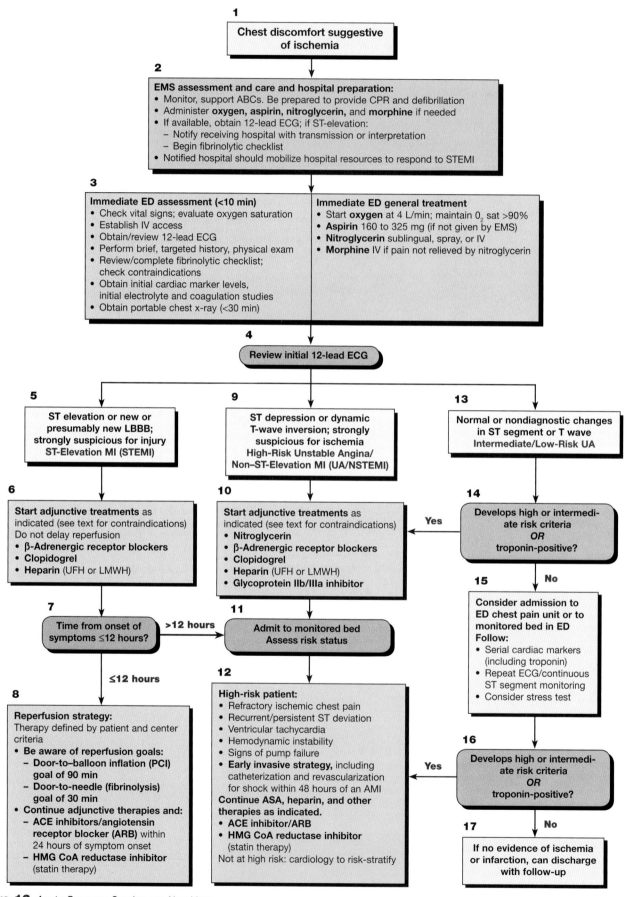

1
Chest discomfort suggestive of ischemia

2
EMS assessment and care and hospital preparation:
- Monitor, support ABCs. Be prepared to provide CPR and defibrillation
- Administer **oxygen, aspirin, nitroglycerin,** and **morphine** if needed
- If available, obtain 12-lead ECG; if ST-elevation:
  – Notify receiving hospital with transmission or interpretation
  – Begin fibrinolytic checklist
- Notified hospital should mobilize hospital resources to respond to STEMI

3
Immediate ED assessment (<10 min)
- Check vital signs; evaluate oxygen saturation
- Establish IV access
- Obtain/review 12-lead ECG
- Perform brief, targeted history, physical exam
- Review/complete fibrinolytic checklist; check contraindications
- Obtain initial cardiac marker levels, initial electrolyte and coagulation studies
- Obtain portable chest x-ray (<30 min)

Immediate ED general treatment
- Start **oxygen** at 4 L/min; maintain 0₂ sat >90%
- **Aspirin** 160 to 325 mg (if not given by EMS)
- **Nitroglycerin** sublingual, spray, or IV
- **Morphine** IV if pain not relieved by nitroglycerin

4
Review initial 12-lead ECG

5
ST elevation or new or presumably new LBBB; strongly suspicious for injury ST-Elevation MI (STEMI)

9
ST depression or dynamic T-wave inversion; strongly suspicious for ischemia High-Risk Unstable Angina/ Non–ST-Elevation MI (UA/NSTEMI)

13
Normal or nondiagnostic changes in ST segment or T wave Intermediate/Low-Risk UA

6
Start adjunctive treatments as indicated (see text for contraindications) Do not delay reperfusion
- **β-Adrenergic receptor blockers**
- **Clopidogrel**
- **Heparin** (UFH or LMWH)

10
Start adjunctive treatments as indicated (see text for contraindications)
- **Nitroglycerin**
- **β-Adrenergic receptor blockers**
- **Clopidogrel**
- **Heparin** (UFH or LMWH)
- **Glycoprotein IIb/IIIa inhibitor**

14
Develops high or intermediate risk criteria OR troponin-positive?

Yes → (to 10)

No ↓

7
Time from onset of symptoms ≤12 hours?

>12 hours →

11
Admit to monitored bed Assess risk status

≤12 hours ↓

15
Consider admission to ED chest pain unit or to monitored bed in ED Follow:
- Serial cardiac markers (including troponin)
- Repeat ECG/continuous ST segment monitoring
- Consider stress test

8
Reperfusion strategy:
Therapy defined by patient and center criteria
- **Be aware of reperfusion goals:**
  – Door-to–balloon inflation (PCI) goal of 90 min
  – Door-to-needle (fibrinolysis) goal of 30 min
- Continue adjunctive therapies and:
  – **ACE inhibitors/angiotensin receptor blocker (ARB)** within 24 hours of symptom onset
  – **HMG CoA reductase inhibitor** (statin therapy)

12
High-risk patient:
- Refractory ischemic chest pain
- Recurrent/persistent ST deviation
- Ventricular tachycardia
- Hemodynamic instability
- Signs of pump failure
- **Early invasive strategy,** including catheterization and revascularization for shock within 48 hours of an AMI
Continue ASA, heparin, and other therapies as indicated.
- **ACE inhibitor/ARB**
- **HMG CoA reductase inhibitor** (statin therapy)
Not at high risk: cardiology to risk-stratify

16
Develops high or intermediate risk criteria OR troponin-positive?

Yes → (to 12)

No ↓

17
If no evidence of ischemia or infarction, can discharge with follow-up

Figure 12. Acute Coronary Syndromes Algorithm.

Starting With Dispatch

All dispatchers and EMS providers must be trained to recognize symptoms of ACS and its complications. Dispatchers, when authorized by medical control or protocol, should tell patients with no history of aspirin allergy or signs of active or recent gastrointestinal (GI) bleeding to chew an aspirin (160 to 325 mg) while waiting for EMS providers to arrive.

EMS Assessment, Care, and Hospital Preparation (Box 2)

Introduction

EMS assessment, care, and hospital preparation are outlined in Box 2. EMS responders may perform the following assessments and actions during the stabilization, triage, and transport of the patient to an appropriate facility:

- Monitor and support ABCs
- Administer oxygen, aspirin, nitroglycerin, and possibly morphine
- Obtain a 12-lead ECG; interpret or transmit for interpretation
- Complete a fibrinolytic checklist if indicated
- Provide prearrival notification to the receiving facility

Monitor and Support ABCs

Monitoring and support of ABCs includes

- Monitoring vital signs and cardiac rhythm
- Being prepared to provide CPR
- Using a defibrillator if needed

Administer Oxygen and Drugs

The following may be administered as indicated:

- Oxygen
- Aspirin
- Nitroglycerin
- Morphine

Providers should be familiar with the actions, indications, cautions, and treatment of side effects.

Oxygen

EMS providers may administer **oxygen** to all patients under evaluation for ACS. Experimental studies have shown that oxygen administration can reduce ST-segment elevation in anterior infarction. It is difficult, however, to document the effects of oxygen on morbidity or mortality. Based largely on consensus opinion, it is reasonable to administer oxygen for about the first 6 hours of therapy. After this time there is no clinical benefit for continued administration except in certain circumstances including

- Patients with continuing/recurrent chest discomfort or hemodynamic instability
- Patients with overt pulmonary congestion
- Patients with oxygen saturation <90%

Aspirin

If the patient has not taken **aspirin** and has no history of aspirin allergy and no evidence of recent GI bleeding, give the patient aspirin (160 to 325 mg) to chew. In the initial hours of an ACS, aspirin is absorbed better when chewed than when swallowed, particularly if morphine has been given. Use rectal ASA suppositories for patients with nausea or vomiting or with active peptic ulcer disease or other disorders of the upper GI tract.

Nitroglycerin

Give the patient up to 3 sublingual *nitroglycerin* tablets (or spray "doses") if no contra-indications, at intervals of 3 to 5 minutes for ongoing symptoms if permitted by medical control. Administer nitroglycerin only if the patient remains hemodynamically stable: systolic blood pressure greater than 90 mm Hg or no lower than 30 mm Hg below baseline (if known) and heart rate 50 to 100/min.

Nitroglycerin is a venodilator and needs to be used cautiously or not at all in patients with inadequate ventricular preload. These situations include

- **Inferior MI and RV infarction.** Use nitroglycerin with caution in patients with inferior wall MI with possible right ventricular (RV) involvement. Patients with acute RV infarction and dysfunction are very dependent on maintenance of RV filling pressures to maintain cardiac output and blood pressure. Nitrates and other vasodilators are contraindicated in these patients.
- **Hypotension, bradycardia, or tachycardia.** Avoid use of nitroglycerin in patients with hypotension (systolic BP<90 mm Hg), marked bradycardia (<50 bpm), or tachycardia.
- **Recent phosphodiesterase inhibitor use (eg, Viagra).** Avoid the use of nitroglycerin if it is suspected or known that the patient has taken sildenafil or vardenafil within the previous 24 hours or tadalafil within 48 hours. Nitrates may cause severe hypotension refractory to vasopressor agents.

Morphine

Give *morphine* for chest pain that is unresponsive to sublingual or spray nitroglycerin if authorized by protocol or medical control.

Morphine is an important treatment for ACS because of the following:

- Produces central nervous system analgesia, which reduces the adverse effects of neurohumoral activation, catecholamine release, and heightened myocardial oxygen demand
- Produces venodilation, which reduces left ventricular (LV) preload and oxygen requirements
- Decreases systemic vascular resistance, thereby reducing LV afterload
- Helps redistribute blood volume in patients with acute pulmonary edema

Remember, morphine is a venodilator. Like nitroglycerin, use morphine with caution in patients who may be preload dependent. If hypotension develops, administer fluids as a first line of therapy.

Obtain a 12-Lead ECG

EMS providers should obtain a 12-lead ECG if available. The *2005 AHA Guidelines for CPR and ECC* recommends out-of-hospital 12-lead ECG diagnostic programs in urban and suburban EMS systems.

EMS Action	Recommendation
12-lead ECG if available	The routine use of 12-lead out-of-hospital ECGs is recommended for patients with signs and symptoms of ACS.
Prearrival hospital notification for STEMI	Prearrival notification of the ED shortens the time to treatment and speeds reperfusion therapy with fibrinolytics or PCI, or both.
Fibrinolytic checklist* if appropriate	If STEMI is identified on the 12-lead ECG, complete a fibrinolytic checklist if appropriate.

*See the student CD for a sample fibrinolytic checklist.

Provide Prearrival Information to Receiving Facility

Time is critical for myocardial salvage in a STEMI patient. EMS notification to the receiving ED can help facilitate early perfusion therapy with fibrinolytics or PCI, or both, as described above. Prior notification of the receiving hospital speeds the diagnosis and shortens the time to reperfusion therapy; reductions of 10 to 60 minutes have been achieved in clinical studies. Prior notification may reduce mortality and minimize myocardial injury.

Immediate ED Assessment and Treatment (Box 3)

Introduction

Upon arrival at the ED, the potential ACS patient should be quickly evaluated. Within the first 10 minutes, obtain a 12-lead ECG (if not already performed before arrival) and assess the patient.

> *The 12-lead ECG is at the center of the decision pathway in the management of ischemic chest pain and is the only means of identifying STEMI.*

The targeted evaluation should focus on chest discomfort, signs and symptoms of heart failure, cardiac history, risk factors for ACS, and historical features that may preclude the use of fibrinolytics. For the patient with STEMI, the goals of reperfusion are to give fibrinolytics within 30 minutes of arrival or provide PCI within 90 minutes of arrival.

Patients with STEMI are candidates for rapid reperfusion. How to measure the ST-segment deviation is shown in Figure 13.

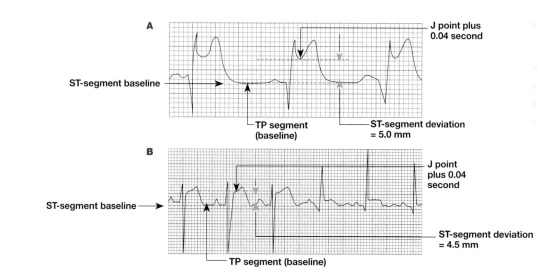

Figure 13. How to measure ST-segment deviation. **A,** Inferior MI. ST segment has no low point (it is coved or concave). **B,** Anterior MI.

Patient Assessment <10 Minutes (Box 3a)

Assessment of the patient in the first 10 minutes should include the following:

- Check vital signs and evaluate oxygen saturation.
- Establish IV access.
- Obtain and review 12-lead ECG.
- Take a brief focused history and perform a physical exam.
- Complete the fibrinolytic checklist and check for contraindications.
- Obtain a blood sample to evaluate initial cardiac marker levels, electrolytes, and coagulation.
- Obtain and review portable chest x-ray (less than 30 minutes after patient's arrival in ED). Should not delay fibrinolytic therapy for STEMI.

Note: Results of cardiac markers, chest x-ray and laboratory studies should not delay reperfusion therapy unless clinically necessary, eg, suspicion of aortic dissection, coagulopathy.

Patient General Treatment (Box 3b)

Unless allergies or contraindications exist, 4 agents are routinely recommended for treatment of patients with ischemic-type chest pain:

- Oxygen
- Aspirin
- Nitroglycerin
- Morphine

Because these agents may have been given out of hospital, administer initial or supplemental doses as indicated. (See the discussion of these drugs in the previous section "EMS Assessment, Care, and Hospital Preparation.")

Critical Concepts:

Oxygen, Aspirin, Nitrates, Morphine

Unless contraindicated, initial therapy with oxygen, aspirin, nitrates and (if indicated) morphine is recommended for all patients suspected of having ischemic chest discomfort.

The major contraindication to nitroglycerin and morphine is hypotension, including hypotension from an RV infarction. The major contraindications to aspirin are true aspirin allergy and active or recent GI bleeding.

Classify Patients According to ST-Segment Deviation (Boxes 5, 9, 13)

Classify Into 3 Groups Based on ST-Segment Deviation

Review the initial 12-Lead ECG (Box 4) and classify patients into 1 of the 3 following clinical groups (Boxes 5, 9, 13):

General Group	Description
STEMI	ST elevation
High-risk UA/NSTEMI	ST depression or dynamic T-wave inversion
Intermediate/low risk UA	Normal or nondiagnostic ECG

1. ***ST-segment elevation myocardial infarction*** (STEMI) is characterized by ST-segment elevation greater than 1 mm (0.1 mV) in 2 or more contiguous precordial leads or 2 or more adjacent limb leads or by new or presumed new left bundle branch block (LBBB).

2. ***High-risk unstable angina (UA) /Non–ST-segment elevation myocardial infarction (NSTEMI)*** is characterized by ischemic ST-segment depression of 0.5 mm (0.05 mV) or greater or dynamic T-wave inversion with pain or discomfort. Nonpersistent or transient ST elevation of 0.5 mm or greater for less than 20 minutes is also included in this category.

3. ***Intermediate or low risk unstable angina (UA)*** is characterized by normal or nondiagnostic changes in ST segment or T wave that are inconclusive and require further risk stratification. This classification includes patients with normal ECGs and those with ST-segment deviation in either direction of less than 0.5 mm (0.05 mV) or T-wave inversion of 2 mm or 0.2 mV or less. Serial cardiac studies and functional testing are appropriate. Note that additional information (troponin) may place the patient into a higher risk after initial classification.

The ECG classification of ischemic syndromes is not meant to be exclusive. A small percentage of patients with normal ECGs may be found to have MI, for example. If the initial ECG is nondiagnostic and clinical circumstances indicate (eg, ongoing chest discomfort), repeat the ECG.

STEMI (Boxes 5-8)

Introduction

Patients with STEMI usually have complete occlusion of an epicardial coronary artery.

> **The mainstay of treatment for STEMI is early reperfusion therapy achieved with fibrinolytics or primary PCI.**

Reperfusion therapy for STEMI is perhaps the most important advancement in treatment of cardiovascular disease in recent years. Early fibrinolytic therapy or direct catheter-based reperfusion has been established as a standard of care for patients with STEMI who present within 12 hours of onset of symptoms with no contraindications. Reperfusion therapy reduces mortality and saves heart muscle. The shorter the time to reperfusion, the greater the benefit. A 47% reduction in mortality was noted when fibrinolytic therapy was provided in the first hour after onset of symptoms.

Early Reperfusion Therapy

Rapidly identify patients with STEMI and quickly screen them for indications and contra-indications to fibrinolytic therapy using a fibrinolytic checklist if appropriate.

The first qualified physician who encounters a patient with STEMI should interpret or confirm the 12-lead ECG, determine the risk/benefit of reperfusion therapy, and direct the administration of fibrinolytic therapy or implementation of PCI. Early activation of PCI may occur with established protocols. The following time frames are recommended:

- If the patient meets the criteria for **fibrinolytic therapy**, an ED door-to-needle time (needle time is the beginning of infusion of a fibrinolytic agent) of 30 minutes or less is desired.
- For **PCI**, an ED door-to–balloon inflation time of 90 minutes or less is desired.

Adjunctive treatments may also be indicated.

Use of Fibrinolytic Therapy

A fibrinolytic agent or "clot-buster" is administered to patients with more than 1 mm ST-segment elevation in 2 anatomically contiguous leads (eg, leads 3, aVF; leads V_3, V_4; leads 1 and aVL) without contraindications. Fibrin-specific agents are effective in achieving normal flow in about 50% of patients given these drugs. Examples of fibrin-specific drugs are tissue plasminogen activator (tPA), reteplase, and tenecteplase. Streptokinase was the first fibrinolytic used widely, but it is not fibrin specific. It is still the most common agent used worldwide for acute STEMI reperfusion therapy.

Considerations for the use of fibrinolytic therapy are as follows:

- In the absence of contraindications and in the presence of a favorable risk-benefit ratio, fibrinolytic therapy is one option for reperfusion in patients with STEMI and *onset of symptoms within 12 hours of presentation* and qualifying ECG findings.
- In the absence of contraindications, it is also reasonable to give fibrinolytics to patients with *onset of symptoms within the prior 12 hours* and ECG findings consistent with true posterior MI. Experienced providers will recognize this as a condition where ST-segment depression in the early precordial leads is equivalent to ST-segment elevation in others. When these changes are associated with other ECG findings, it is suggestive of a "STEMI" on the posterior wall of the heart.
- Fibrinolytics are generally not recommended for patients presenting *more than 12 hours after onset of symptoms*. But they may be considered if ischemic chest pain continues with persistent ST-segment elevation of more than 1 mm in 2 or more contiguous chest or limb leads.
- Do not give fibrinolytics to patients who present *more than 24 hours after the onset of symptoms* or patients with ST-segment depression unless a true posterior MI is suspected.

Use of PCI

The most commonly used form of PCI is coronary angioplasty with or without stent placement. *Primary PCI* is used as an alternative to fibrinolytics. *Rescue PCI* is used early after fibrinolytics in patients who may have persistent occlusion of the infarct artery (failure to reperfuse with fibrinolytics). PCI has been shown to be superior to fibrinolysis in the combined end points of death, stroke, and reinfarction in many studies for patients presenting between 3 and 12 hours after onset. But these results have been achieved in experienced medical settings with skilled providers (performing more than 75 PCIs per year) at a skilled PCI facility (performing more than 200 PCIs for STEMI with cardiac surgery capabilities).

Considerations for the use of PCI includes the following:

- At the time of publication of the *2005 AHA Guidelines for CPR and ECC*, primary PCI was preferred in patients with STEMI and *symptom duration of more than 3 hours and less than 12 hours* if skilled personnel ensured that door-to-balloon time was within 90 minutes or that the difference in time between administration of fibrinolytics versus inflation of the PCI balloon was within 60 minutes.

- PCI is also preferred in patients with contraindications to fibrinolytics and is reasonable in patients with cardiogenic shock or heart failure complicating MI.

- In patients with STEMI who present *3 hours or less from onset of symptoms*, treatment is more time sensitive, and there is inadequate research to recommend one treatment over the other. In these "early presenters," any possible benefit from primary PCI will be lost in prolonged transfers.

Adjunctive Treatments

Other drugs are useful in addition to oxygen, sublingual or spray nitroglycerin, aspirin, morphine, and fibrinolytic therapy. These include

- IV nitroglycerin
- Heparin
- Clopidogrel
- β-blockers
- Angiotensin-converting enzyme (ACE) inhibitors
- HMG coenzyme inhibitor therapy (statin)

IV nitroglycerin and heparin are commonly used early in the management of patients with STEMI. These agents are briefly discussed below. We will not review the use of β-blockers, ACE inhibitors, and statin therapy in STEMI. Use of these agents requires additional risk stratification skills and a detailed knowledge of the spectrum of ACS and, in some instances, continuing knowledge of the results of clinical trials.

Intravenous Nitroglycerin

Routine use of IV nitroglycerin is not indicated and has not been shown to significantly reduce mortality in STEMI. IV nitroglycerin is indicated and used widely in ischemic syndromes. It is preferred over topical or long-acting forms because it can be titrated in a patient with potentially unstable hemodynamics and ventricular function.

Indications for initiation of IV nitroglycerin in STEMI are

- Recurrent or continuing chest discomfort unresponsive to SL or spray nitroglycerin and morphine
- Pulmonary edema complicating STEMI
- Hypertension complicating STEMI

Treatment goals using IV nitroglycerin are as follows:

Treatment Goal	Management
Relief of ischemic chest discomfort	• Titrate to effect • Keep SBP >90 mm Hg • Limit drop in SBP to 30 mm Hg below baseline in hypertensive patients
Improvement in pulmonary edema and hypertension	• Titrate to effect • Limit drop in SBP to 10% of baseline in normotensive patients • Limit drop in SBP to 30 mm Hg below baseline in hypertensive patients

Heparin

Heparin administration is routinely given as an adjunct for PCI and fibrinolytic therapy with fibrin-specific agents (tPA, reteplase, tenecteplase). It is also indicated in other specific high-risk situations, such as LV mural thrombus, atrial fibrillation, and prophylaxis for pulmonary thromboembolism in patients with prolonged bed rest and heart failure complicating MI. If you use these drugs you must be familiar with dosing schedules for specific clinical strategies.

 Specific dosing of UFH and LMWH is included in the drug section of the student CD.

> *The inappropriate dosing and monitoring of heparin therapy has caused excess intracerebral bleeding and major hemorrhage in STEMI patients. Providers using heparin need to know the indications, dosing, and use in the specific ACS categories.*
>
> *The dosing, use, and duration have been derived from use in clinical trials. Specific patients may require dose modification. See the ECC Handbook for weight-based dosing guidelines, intervals for administration, and adjustment (if needed) in renal function. See ACC/AHA Guidelines for detailed discussion in specific categories.*

Bradycardia Case

Introduction

This case discusses assessment and management of a *patient with symptomatic bradycardia*. The cornerstones of managing bradycardia are to

- Differentiate between signs and symptoms that are caused by the slow rate versus those that are unrelated
- Correctly diagnose the presence and type of atrioventricular (AV) block
- Use atropine when appropriate as the drug intervention of first choice
- Decide when to start transcutaneous pacing (TCP)
- Decide when to start epinephrine or dopamine to maintain heart rate and blood pressure

In addition, you must know the techniques and cautions for using TCP.

Learning Objectives

By the end of this case you will be able to

1. Recognize symptomatic bradycardia and recall its signs, symptoms, causes, and treatment
2. Determine whether signs and symptoms are caused by bradycardia or by another condition
3. Correctly identify and recall the intervention sequence for second-degree and third-degree AV blocks and why it is important to tell the difference between them
4. Determine when to start TCP
5. Recall indications and doses of drugs for treatment of bradycardia, including atropine, dopamine, and epinephrine

2° Type I/II – below AV Node.
3°

c̄ pacer – ck for capture

Rhythms for Bradycardia

This case involves these ECG rhythms:

- Sinus bradycardia
- First-degree AV block
- Second-degree AV block
  - Type I (Wenckebach/Mobitz I)
  - Type II (Mobitz II)
- Third-degree AV block

You should know the major AV blocks because important treatment decisions are based on the type of block present (see Figure 14). Complete AV block is generally the most important and clinically significant degree of block. Also, complete or third-degree AV block is the degree of block most likely to cause cardiovascular collapse and require immediate pacing. *Recognition of a symptomatic bradycardia due to AV block is a primary goal.* Recognition of the type of AV block is a secondary goal.

Drugs for Bradycardia

This case involves these drugs:

- Atropine
- Dopamine (infusion)
- Epinephrine (infusion)

Description of Bradycardia

Definitions

Definitions used in this case are as follows:

Term	Definition
Bradyarrhythmia or bradycardia*	Any rhythm disorder with a heart rate less than 60 beats per minute (bpm)—eg, third-degree AV block—or sinus bradycardia
Symptomatic bradyarrhythmia	Signs and symptoms that are due to the slow heart rate

*For purposes of this case we will use the term *bradycardia* interchangeably with *bradyarrhythmia* unless specifically defined.

Symptomatic Bradycardia

Sinus bradycardia may have multiple causes. Some are physiologic and require no assessment or therapy. For example, a well-trained athlete may have a heart rate in the 40 to 50 bpm range or occasionally lower.

In contrast, some patients have heart rates in the normal sinus range, but these heart rates are inappropriate or insufficient for them. This is called a *functional* or *relative* bradycardia. For example, a heart rate of 70 bpm is too slow for a patient in cardiogenic or septic shock.

This case will focus on the patient with a bradycardia and heart rate <60 bpm. Key to the case management is the determination of symptoms or signs due to the decreased heart rate. A symptomatic bradycardia exists clinically when 3 criteria are present:

1. The heart rate is slow.
2. The patient has symptoms.
3. The symptoms are due to the slow heart rate.

A

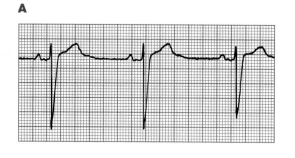

B

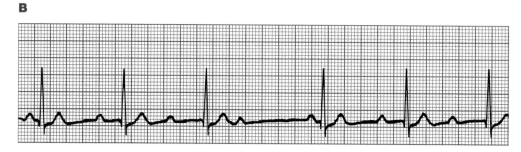

C

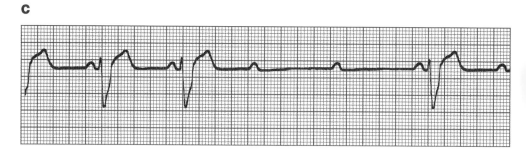

D

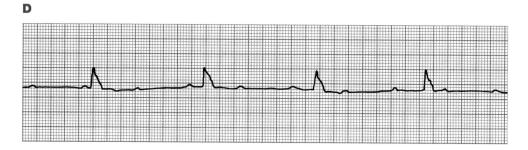

E

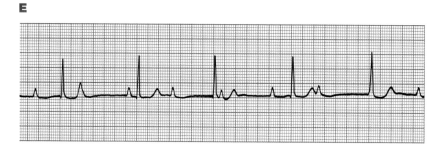

Figure 14. Examples of atrioventricular block (AV block). **A,** Sinus bradycardia with borderline first-degree AV block. **B,** Second-degree AV block type I. **C,** Second-degree AV block type II. **D,** Complete AV block with a ventricular escape pacemaker (wide QRS: 0.12 to 0.14 sec). **E,** Third-degree AV block with a junctional escape pacemaker (narrow QRS: <0.12).

Signs and Symptoms

You must perform a focused history and physical examination to identify symptomatic bradycardia (symptoms and signs).

Symptoms include chest discomfort or pain, shortness of breath, decreased level of consciousness, weakness, fatigue, lightheadedness, dizziness, and presyncope or syncope.

Signs include hypotension; drop in blood pressure upon standing (orthostatic hypotension); diaphoresis; pulmonary congestion on physical examination or chest x-ray; frank congestive heart failure or pulmonary edema; and bradycardia-related (escape), frequent premature ventricular complexes (PVCs) or VT.

Managing Bradycardia: the ACLS Bradycardia Algorithm

Overview of the Algorithm

The ACLS Bradycardia Algorithm (Figure 15) outlines the steps for assessment and management of a patient presenting with symptomatic bradycardia. Implementation of this algorithm begins with the identification of bradycardia (Box 1). First steps include the components of the BLS Primary Survey and the ACLS Secondary Survey, such as supporting ABCs, giving oxygen, monitoring the rhythm and vital signs, and establishing IV access (Box 2). In Differential Diagnosis you determine if the patient has signs or symptoms of poor perfusion and if these are caused by the bradycardia (Box 3).

The primary decision point in the algorithm is the determination of adequate perfusion. If the patient has adequate perfusion, you observe and monitor (Box 4A). If the patient has poor perfusion, you prepare for TCP and consider administration of drugs (Box 4). If indicated, you prepare for transvenous pacing, search for and treat contributing causes, and seek expert consultation (Box 5).

The treatment sequence in the algorithm is determined by the severity of the patient's condition. You may need to implement multiple interventions simultaneously. If pulseless arrest develops, go to the Pulseless Arrest Algorithm.

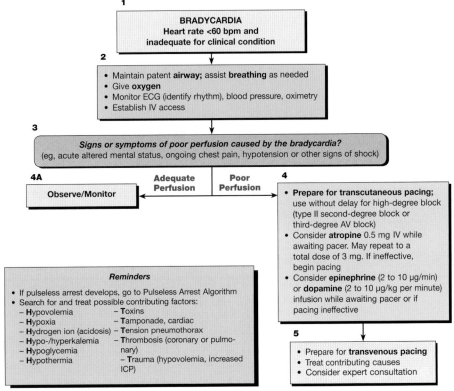

Figure 15. Bradycardia Algorithm.

Application of the Bradycardia Algorithm

Introduction	In this case you have a patient presenting with symptoms of bradycardia. You conduct appropriate assessment and interventions as outlined in the Bradycardia Algorithm. At the same time you are searching for and treating possible contributing factors.

Identification of Bradycardia (Box 1)

Identify whether the bradycardia is
- Present by definition, ie, heart rate <60 bpm
- Inadequate for the patient's condition (functional or relative)

A *bradycardia* is generally defined as a heart rate <60 bpm. But in many people, particularly trained athletes, slow heart rate produces effective systemic perfusion.

In *relative bradycardia* the pulse rate is less than expected in relation to the underlying condition or cause.

Primary and Secondary Surveys (Box 2)

Next, perform the BLS Primary Survey and the ACLS Secondary Survey, including the following:

A	Maintain patent airway.
B	Assist breathing as needed; give oxygen; monitor oxygen saturation.
C	Monitor blood pressure and heart rate; obtain and review 12-lead ECG; establish IV access.
D	Conduct a problem-focused history and physical examination; search for and treat possible contributing factors.

Are Signs or Symptoms Caused by Bradycardia? (Box 3)

Box 3 prompts you to consider if the signs or symptoms of poor perfusion are caused by the bradycardia.

The key clinical questions are
- Are there "serious" signs or symptoms?
- Are the signs and symptoms related to the slow heart rate?

Look for adverse signs and symptoms of the bradycardia:
- Symptoms (eg, chest pain, shortness of breath, decreased level of consciousness, weakness, fatigue, lightheadedness, dizziness, and presyncope or syncope)
- Signs (eg, hypotension, congestive heart failure, ventricular arrhythmias related to the bradycardia)

Sometimes the "symptom" is not due to the bradycardia. For example, hypotension associated with bradycardia may be due to myocardial dysfunction rather than to the bradycardia. Keep this in mind when you reassess the patient's response to treatment.

Critical Concepts: Bradycardia

The key clinical question is whether the bradycardia is causing the patient's symptoms or some other illness is causing the bradycardia.

Decision Point: Adequate Perfusion?

You must now decide if the patient's perfusion is adequate or poor.
- If the patient has ***adequate perfusion,*** observe and monitor (Box 4A).
- If the patient has ***poor perfusion,*** proceed to Box 4.

Treatment Sequence Summary (Box 4)

If the patient has poor perfusion secondary to bradycardia, the treatment sequence is as follows:

Prepare for transcutaneous pacing	Prepare for and use TCP without delay for high-degree block (eg, Mobitz type II second-degree block or third-degree AV block)
Consider atropine while awaiting pacer	Atropine 0.5 mg IV—may repeat to a total dose of 3 mg
If atropine is ineffective, begin pacing	
Consider epinephrine or dopamine infusion while awaiting pacemaker or if pacing is ineffective	• Epinephrine 2 to 10 µg/min • Dopamine 2 to 10 µg/kg per minute (chronotropic or heart rate dose)

The treatment sequence is determined by the severity of the patient's clinical presentation. For patients with symptomatic bradycardia, move quickly through this sequence. These patients may be "pre–cardiac arrest" and may need multiple interventions simultaneously, such as TCP pending transvenous pacing, IV atropine, and infusion of dopamine or epinephrine. In the absence of immediately reversible causes, atropine is the first-line drug for symptomatic bradycardia.

Treatment Sequence: Pacing

TCP should be started immediately for symptomatic patients who are unstable, particularly those with a high-degree block (Mobitz type II second-degree block or third-degree AV block). TCP is noninvasive and can be performed by ACLS providers.

Start TCP immediately if

- There is no response to atropine
- Atropine is unlikely to be effective or if IV access cannot be quickly established
- The patient is severely symptomatic

Following initiation of pacing, confirm electrical and mechanical capture. Reassess the patient for symptomatic improvement and hemodynamic stability. Give analgesics and sedatives for pain control. Note that many of these drugs may further decrease blood pressure and affect the patient's mental status. Try to identify and correct the cause of the bradycardia.

Some limitations apply. TCP can be painful and may fail to produce effective electrical and mechanical capture. If symptoms are not caused by the bradycardia, pacing may be ineffective despite capture.

If TCP is ineffective (eg, inconsistent capture), prepare for transvenous pacing and obtain expert consultation.

Treatment Sequence: Atropine

In the absence of immediately reversible causes, atropine remains the first-line drug for acute symptomatic bradycardia. Failure to respond to atropine is an indication for TCP, although use of second-line drugs such as dopamine and epinephrine may be successful.

For bradycardia give atropine 0.5 mg IV every 3 to 5 minutes to a total dose of 0.04 mg/kg (maximum total dose of 3 mg). Atropine doses of less than 0.5 mg may paradoxically result in further slowing of the heart rate.

Use atropine cautiously in the presence of acute coronary ischemia or MI. An atropine-mediated increase in heart rate may worsen ischemia or increase infarct size.

Do not rely on atropine in Mobitz type II second-degree or third-degree AV block or in patients with third-degree AV block with a new wide QRS complex. Hemodynamically unstable and clinically deteriorating patients require immediate pacing. All other awake patients should have sedation before pacing.

Foundation Facts:

Sedation and Pacing

Most awake patients should be given sedation before pacing. If the patient is in cardio-vascular collapse or rapidly deteriorating, it may be necessary to start pacing without prior sedation, particularly if drugs for sedation are not immediately available. The clinician must evaluate the need for sedation in light of the patient's condition and need for immediate pacing. A review of the drugs used is beyond the scope of the ACLS Provider Course. The general approach could include the following:

- Give parenteral benzodiazepine for anxiety and muscle contractions
- Give a parenteral narcotic for analgesia
- Obtain expert consultation for transvenous pacing

Treatment Sequence: Epinephrine, Dopamine

For bradycardia unresponsive to atropine, consider a titrated epinephrine or dopamine infusion as a temporizing measure until pacing is started. To simplify the algorithm, we have listed epinephrine and dopamine as alternatives to consider because they are both widely available.

An epinephrine infusion may be given to patients with symptomatic bradycardia or hypotension after atropine or TCP failure. Begin the infusion at a dose of 2 to 10 µg/min and titrate to patient response.

Dopamine hydrochloride has both α-adrenergic and β-adrenergic actions. Begin the dopamine infusion at 2 to 10 µg/kg per minute and titrate to patient response. Dopamine can be added to epinephrine or given alone. Assess intravascular volume and support as needed. Note that the heart rate (chronotropic) dose of dopamine will likely be lower than the vasoconstrictor (inotropic) dose range.

Next Actions (Box 5)

After consideration of the treatment sequence in Box 4, you may need to

- Prepare the patient for transvenous pacing
- Treat the contributing causes of the bradycardia
- Consider expert consultation—but do not delay treatment if the patient is unstable or potentially unstable.

Transcutaneous Pacing (TCP)

Introduction	Transcutaneous pacing (TCP) is the treatment of choice when a patient has a symptomatic bradycardia with signs of poor perfusion.

A variety of devices can pace the heart by delivering an electrical stimulus, causing electrical depolarization and subsequent cardiac contraction. TCP delivers pacing impulses to the heart through the skin by using cutaneous electrodes. Most manufacturers have added a pacing mode to manual defibrillators.

The ability to perform TCP is now often as close as the nearest defibrillator. Providers need to know the indications, techniques, and hazards for using TCP.

Indications

Indications for TCP are as follows:

- Hemodynamically unstable bradycardia (eg, blood pressure changes, altered mental status, angina, pulmonary edema)
- Unstable clinical condition that is likely due to the bradycardia
- For pacing readiness in the setting of AMI as follows:
  - Symptomatic sinus bradycardia
  - Mobitz type II second-degree AV block
  - Third-degree AV block
  - New left, right, or alternating bundle branch block or bifascicular block
- Bradycardia with symptomatic ventricular escape rhythms
- Overdrive pacing of tachycardias refractory to drug therapy or electrical cardioversion

Precautions

Precautions for TCP are as follows:

- TCP is contraindicated in severe hypothermia and is not recommended for asystole.
- Conscious patients require analgesia for discomfort unless delay for sedation will cause/contribute to deterioration.
- Do not assess the carotid pulse to confirm mechanical capture; electrical stimulation causes muscular jerking that may mimic the carotid pulse.

Technique

Perform TCP by following these steps:

Step	Action
1	Place pacing electrodes on the chest per package instructions.
2	Turn the pacer ON.
3	Set the demand rate to approximately 60/min. This rate can be adjusted up or down (based on patient clinical response) once pacing is established.
4	Set the current milliamperes (mA) output 2 mA above the dose at which consistent capture is observed (safety margin).

External pacemakers have either *fixed* rates (asynchronous mode) or *demand* rates.

Recommendations for Use of TCP

Use TCP for the following:

- Hemodynamically significant (symptomatic) bradyarrhythmia
- Bradycardia with escape rhythms
- Standby pacing

Assess Response to Treatment

Rather than target a precise heart rate, the goal of therapy is to ensure improvement in clinical status (ie, signs and symptoms related to the bradycardia). Signs of hemodynamic impairment include hypotension, change in mental status, angina, pulmonary edema, seizures, syncope, or other signs of shock related to the bradycardia. Start pacing at a rate of about 60/min. Once pacing is initiated, adjust the rate based on the patient's clinical response. Most patients will improve with a rate of 60/min to 70/min if the symptoms are primarily due to the bradycardia.

Consider giving atropine before pacing in mildly symptomatic patients. But do not delay pacing for unstable patients, particularly those with high-degree AV block. Atropine may increase heart rate, improve hemodynamics, and eliminate the need for pacing. If atropine is ineffective or likely to be ineffective or if establishment of IV access or atropine administration is delayed, begin pacing as soon as it is available.

Patients with acute ischemia (ACS) should be paced at the lowest heart rate that allows clinical stability. Higher heart rates can worsen ischemia because heart rate is a major determinate of myocardial oxygen demand. Ischemia, in turn, can precipitate arrhythmias.

If pacing is not immediately available and the symptomatic bradycardia is unresponsive to atropine, consider catecholamine use in doses that stimulate heart rate (chronotropic doses):

- Epinephrine: initiate at 2 to 10 µg/min and titrate to patient response
- Dopamine: initiate at 2 to 10 µg/kg per minute and titrate to patient response.

Bradycardia With Escape Rhythms

A bradycardia may lead to bradycardia-dependent ventricular rhythms. When the heart rate falls, an electrically unstable ventricular area may "escape" suppression by higher and faster pacemakers (eg, sinus node), especially in the setting of acute ischemia. These ventricular rhythms often fail to respond to drugs. With severe bradycardia some patients will develop a wide-complex ventricular beats that can precipitate VT or VF. Pacing may increase the heart rate and eliminate bradycardia-dependent ventricular rhythms. However, an accelerated idioventricular rhythm (sometimes called AIVR) may occur in the setting of inferior wall MI. This rhythm is usually stable and does not require pacing.

Patients with ventricular escape rhythms may have normal myocardium with disturbed conduction. After correction of electrolyte abnormalities or acidosis, rapid pacing can stimulate effective myocardial contractions until the conduction system recovers.

Standby Pacing

Several bradycardic rhythms in ACS are caused by acute ischemia of conduction tissue and pacing centers. Patients who are clinically stable may decompensate suddenly or become unstable over minutes to hours from worsening conduction abnormalities. These bradycardias may deteriorate to complete AV block and cardiovascular collapse.

Place TCP electrodes in anticipation of clinical deterioration in patients with acute myocardial ischemia or infarction associated with the following rhythms:

- Symptomatic sinus node dysfunction with severe and symptomatic sinus bradycardia
- Asymptomatic Mobitz type II second-degree AV block
- Asymptomatic third-degree AV block
- Newly acquired left, right, or alternating bundle branch block or bifascicular block in the setting of AMI

Unstable Tachycardia Case

Introduction	If you are the team leader in this case, you will conduct the assessment and management of a *patient with a rapid, unstable heart rate*. You must be able to classify the tachycardia and implement appropriate interventions as outlined in the ACLS Tachycardia Algorithm. You will be evaluated on your knowledge of the factors involved in safe and effective synchronized cardioversion as well as your performance of the procedure.
Learning Objectives	By the end of this case you should be able to

1. Recall features of stable and unstable tachycardias
2. Follow the ACLS initial assessment and management recommendations in the Tachycardia Algorithm (Figure 16)
3. Identify the patient as unstable and follow the unstable tachycardia arm of the Tachycardia Algorithm (Figure 16)
4. Recall the energy levels required for electrical cardioversion of different tachycardias and the standard sequence of energy levels for synchronized cardioversion
5. Demonstrate safe and effective cardioversion

Rhythms for Unstable Tachycardia	This case involves these ECG rhythms:

- Atrial fibrillation
- Atrial flutter
- Reentry supraventricular tachycardia (SVT)
- Monomorphic VT
- Polymorphic VT
- Wide-complex tachycardia of uncertain type

Drugs for Unstable Tachycardia	Drugs are not used to manage patients with unstable tachycardia. Immediate cardioversion is recommended. Consider administering sedative drugs in the awake patient. But do not delay immediate cardioversion in the unstable patient.

Approach to Unstable Tachycardia

Introduction	A tachyarrhythmia (rhythm with heart rate >100 bpm) has many potential causes and may be symptomatic or asymptomatic. The key to management of a patient with any tachycardia is to determine whether pulses are present. If pulses are present, determine whether the patient is stable or unstable and then provide treatment based on patient condition and rhythm.

If the tachyarrhythmia is sinus tachycardia, conduct a diligent search for the cause of the tachycardia. Treatment and correction of this cause will improve the signs and symptoms.

Definitions

Definitions used in this case are as follows:

Term	Definition
Tachyarrhythmia, tachycardia*	Heart rate >100 bpm
Symptomatic tachyarrhythmia	Signs and symptoms that are due to the rapid heart rate

*For purposes of this case we will use the term *tachycardia* interchangeably with *tachyarrhythmia*. *Sinus tachycardia* will be specifically indicated.

Pathophysiology of Unstable Tachycardia

Unstable tachycardia exists when the heart rate is too fast for the patient's clinical condition and the excessive heart rate causes symptoms or an unstable condition because the heart is

- *Beating so fast* that cardiac output is reduced; this can cause pulmonary edema, coronary ischemia, and reduced blood flow to vital organs (eg, brain, kidneys)
- *Beating ineffectively* so that coordination between atrium and ventricles or the ventricles themselves reduce cardiac output

Symptoms and Signs

Unstable tachycardia leads to serious signs and symptoms.

Symptoms that may be due to tachycardia include

- Shortness of breath
- Chest pain
- Altered mental status
- Weakness, fatigue, near-fainting (presyncope), syncope

Signs include

- Hypotension
- Ischemic ECG changes
- Pulmonary edema (CHF)
- Poor peripheral perfusion (altered mental status, cool extremities, decreased urine output)

Rapid Recognition Is the Key to Management

The 2 keys to management of patients with unstable tachycardia are

1. Rapid recognition that the patient is *significantly symptomatic* or even *unstable*
2. Rapid recognition that the *signs and symptoms are caused by the tachycardia*

> *You must quickly determine whether the patient's tachycardia is producing hemodynamic instability and serious signs and symptoms or whether the signs and symptoms (eg, the pain and distress of an AMI) are producing the tachycardia.*
>
> This determination can be difficult. In general, heart rates between 100/min and approximately 130/min are usually the result of an underlying process and often represent sinus tachycardia. Heart rates >150/min may be symptomatic; the higher the rate the more likely symptoms are due to the tachycardia. Underlying heart disease or other comorbidities can cause symptoms at lower heart rates.

Severity	Assess for the presence or absence of signs and symptoms and for their severity. Frequent patient assessment is indicated.
Indications for Cardioversion	Rapid identification of symptomatic tachycardia will help you determine whether you should prepare for immediate cardioversion. For example:

- *Sinus tachycardia* is a physiologic response to extrinsic factors that create the need for increased cardiac output. There is usually a high degree of sympathetic tone and neurohormonal factors. Sinus tachycardia will not respond to cardioversion. In fact, if a shock is delivered, the heart rate often increases.
- *Atrial flutter* typically produces a heart rate of approximately 150 bpm (lower rates may be present in patients who have received antiarrhythmic therapy). Atrial flutter at this rate is often stable in the patient without heart or serious systemic disease.
- At rates above 150 bpm, symptoms are often present and cardioversion is often required if the patient is unstable.
- If the patient is seriously ill or has underlying cardiovascular disease, symptoms may be present at lower rates.

You must know when cardioversion is indicated, how to prepare the patient for it (including appropriate medication), and how to switch the defibrillator/monitor to operate as a cardioverter.

Managing Unstable Tachycardia: the ACLS Tachycardia Algorithm

Introduction	The ACLS Tachycardia Algorithm combines several previous ACLS algorithms and simplifies initial management of tachycardia. The key to management of a patient with any tachycardia is to determine whether pulses are present. If pulses are present, determine whether the patient is stable or unstable and then provide treatment based on patient condition and rhythm. If a pulseless tachycardia is present, then manage the patient according to the ACLS Pulseless Arrest Algorithm.

The ACLS Provider Course focuses on the initial parts of the ACLS Tachycardia Algorithm, those boxes that are not printed with screening (screened text appears lighter than regular text). Before proceeding into the screened areas of the algorithm, the ACLS Provider should either be an expert or be able to obtain expert consultation. Actions in boxes that are screened require advanced knowledge of ECG and rhythm interpretation and antiarrhythmic therapy and are intended to be accomplished in the in-hospital setting with expert consultation available.

Overview	The ACLS Tachycardia Algorithm (Figure 16) outlines the steps for assessment and management of a patient presenting with symptomatic tachycardia with pulses. Implementation of this algorithm begins with the identification of tachycardia with pulses (Box 1). If a tachycardia and a pulse are present, perform assessment and management steps guided by the BLS Primary Survey and the ACLS Secondary Survey (Box 2). The key in this assessment is to decide if the tachycardia is stable or unstable (Box 3). Determining if symptoms or signs are present and if these symptoms and signs are due to the tachycardia will direct you to either the stable or unstable branch of the algorithm.

If signs and symptoms persist despite provision of supplementary oxygen and support of airway and circulation and if significant signs or symptoms are due to the tachycardia, then the tachycardia is unstable and immediate cardioversion is indicated (Box 4).

If the patient is stable, you will evaluate the ECG, determine if the QRS complex is wide or narrow and regular or irregular. The treatment of stable tachycardia is presented in the next case.

A precise diagnosis of the rhythm (eg, reentry SVT, atrial flutter) may not be possible at this time.

Foundation Facts:

Serious or Significant Symptoms

Unstable Condition

Intervention is determined by the presence of significant symptoms or by an unstable condition resulting from the tachycardia.*

Serious symptoms and signs include

- Altered mental status
- Ongoing chest discomfort or shortness of breath
- Presyncope or syncope

Unstable patients include those with

- Hypotension
- Signs of shock

*Note: Ventricular rates <150/min usually do not cause serious signs or symptoms.

Summary

Your assessment and management of this patient will be guided by the following key questions presented in the ACLS Tachycardia Algorithm:

- Are symptoms present or absent?
- Is the patient stable or unstable?
- Is the QRS narrow or wide?
- Is the rhythm regular or irregular?

Your answers to these questions will determine the next appropriate steps.

Application of the ACLS Tachycardia Algorithm to the Unstable Patient

Introduction

In this case you have a patient with tachycardia and a pulse. You conduct the steps outlined in the ACLS Tachycardia Algorithm to evaluate and manage the patient.

Primary and Secondary Surveys (Box 2)

Use the BLS Primary Survey and the ACLS Secondary Survey to guide your approach. Evaluate the patient and do the following:

- Support the airway, breathing, and circulation.
- Give oxygen; monitor oxygen saturation.
- Obtain an ECG to identify the rhythm; check blood pressure.
- Identify and treat reversible causes.

If symptoms persist despite support of adequate oxygenation and ventilation, proceed to Box 3.

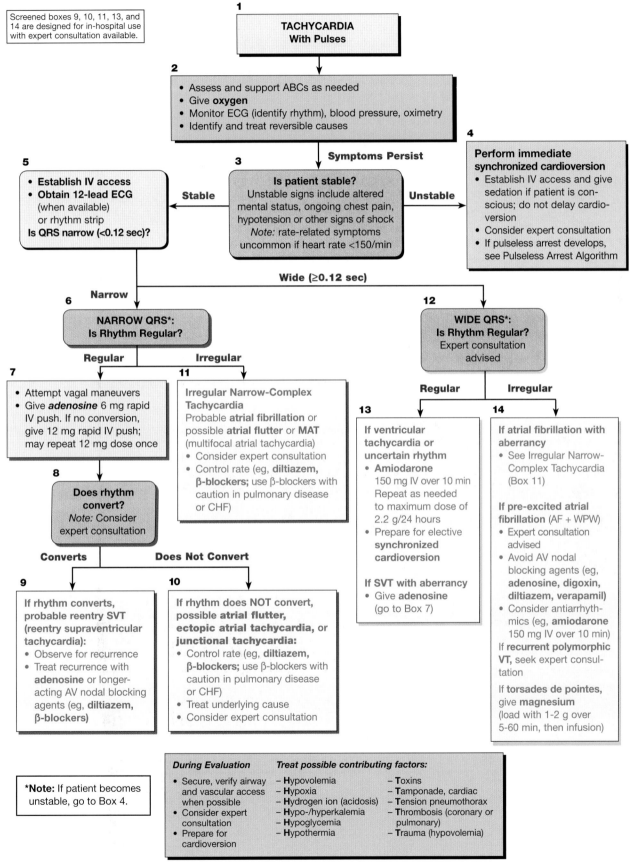

Figure 16. ACLS Tachycardia Algorithm.

Decision Point: Stable or Unstable (Box 3)

Evaluate the patient to determine whether the patient is stable or unstable.

Unstable

If the patient is unstable with signs or symptoms (eg, altered mental status, ongoing chest discomfort or pain, hypotension, or other signs of shock) resulting from the tachycardia, go to Box 4 (perform immediate synchronized cardioversion).

Serious signs and symptoms are unlikely if the ventricular rate is <150/min in patients with a healthy heart. However, if the patient is seriously ill or has significant underlying heart disease or other conditions, symptoms may be present at a lower heart rate.

Stable

If the patient is stable, go to Box 5. Establish IV access (if not already present) and obtain a 12-lead ECG (when available) or rhythm strip to determine if QRS is narrow or wide. We will continue with our discussion of the steps in the algorithm focusing on the stable patient in the Stable Tachycardia Case.

Foundation Facts:

Treatment Based on Type of Tachycardia

You may not always be able to distinguish between supraventricular and ventricular rhythms. Most wide-complex (broad-complex) tachycardias are ventricular in origin (especially if the patient has underlying heart disease or is older). If the patient is pulseless, treat the rhythm as VF and follow the ACLS Pulseless Arrest Algorithm.

If the patient has a wide-complex tachycardia and is unstable, assume it is VT until proven otherwise. The amount of energy required for cardioversion of VT is determined by the morphologic characteristics.

- A regular uniform wide-complex VT is called *monomorphic VT.* If the patient is unstable but has a pulse, do the following:
  - Treat with synchronized cardioversion and an initial shock of 100 J (monophasic waveform)
  - If there is no response to the first shock, increase the dose in a stepwise fashion (200 J, 300 J, 360 J)
- If the patient has *polymorphic VT* and is unstable:
  - Treat as VF with high-energy unsynchronized shocks (eg, defibrillation doses)

If there is any doubt about whether an unstable patient has monomorphic or polymorphic VT, do not delay treatment for further rhythm analysis. Provide high-energy, unsynchronized shocks.

Perform Immediate Synchronized Cardioversion (Box 4)

Establish IV access. Perform immediate synchronized cardioversion.

> Provide sedation to a conscious patient if possible, but **do not delay cardioversion if you think the tachycardia is causing the unstable signs and symptoms or if the patient is clinically deteriorating.**

Consider expert consultation, but do not delay treatment if the patient is unstable or potentially unstable. If the patient is unstable with narrow-complex SVT, give adenosine (if IV access is established) while preparing for synchronized cardioversion. Provide sedation if possible. *But do not delay cardioversion in the extremely unstable patient for administration of adenosine or sedation.*

Consider expert consultation. If pulseless arrest develops, see the Pulseless Arrest Algorithm.

Cardioversion

Introduction

You must know when cardioversion is indicated and what type of shock to administer. Before cardioversion, establish IV access and sedate the responsive patient if possible. But do not delay cardioversion in the unstable or deteriorating patient.

This section discusses the following important concepts about cardioversion:

- Difference between unsynchronized and synchronized shocks
- Potential challenges to delivery of synchronized shocks
- Energy doses for specific rhythms

Unsynchronized vs Synchronized Shocks

Modern defibrillator/cardioverters are capable of delivering 2 types of shocks:

- Unsynchronized shocks
- Synchronized shocks

An *unsynchronized* shock simply means that the electrical shock will be delivered as soon as the operator pushes the SHOCK button to discharge the machine. Thus the shock may fall randomly anywhere within the cardiac cycle. *These shocks should use higher energy levels than synchronized cardioversion.*

Synchronized cardioversion uses a sensor to deliver a shock that is synchronized with a peak of the QRS complex (for example, highest point of the R wave). When this option (the "sync" option) is engaged, the operator presses the SHOCK buttons to deliver a shock. There will likely be a delay before the defibrillator/cardioverter delivers a shock because the device will synchronize shock delivery with the peak of the R wave in the patient's QRS complex. This synchronization may require analysis of several complexes. Synchronization avoids the delivery of a shock during cardiac repolarization (represented on the surface ECG as the T wave), a period of vulnerability in which a shock can precipitate VF. Synchronized cardioversion uses a lower energy level than attempted defibrillation. Low-energy shocks should always be delivered as synchronized shocks to avoid precipitating VF.

Critical Concept:

Low- vs High-Energy Shocks

Low-energy shocks should always be delivered as synchronized shocks. Delivery of low-energy shocks as unsychronized shocks is likely to induce VF. If cardioversion is needed and it is not possible to synchronize a shock (eg, the patient's rhythm is very fast and irregular) use high-energy unsynchronized shocks (defibrillation doses).

Potential Problems with Synchronization

In theory synchronization is simple. The operator pushes the SYNC control on the face of the defibrillator/cardioverter. In practice, however, there are potential problems. For example:

- If the R-wave peaks of a tachycardia are undifferentiated or of low amplitude, the monitor sensors may be unable to identify an R-wave peak and therefore will not deliver the shock.
- Many cardioverters will not synchronize through the hand-held quick-look paddles. An unwary practitioner may try to synchronize—unsuccessfully in that the machine will not discharge—and may not recognize the problem.
- Synchronization can take extra time (eg, if it is necessary to attach electrodes or it the operator is unfamiliar with the equipment).

Recommendations

Below are recommendations for when to use

- Synchronized shocks
- Unsynchronized shocks

When to Use Synchronized Shocks

Synchronized shocks are recommended for

- A patient with symptomatic stable tachycardia
- A patient with unstable tachycardia with pulses

When to Use Unsynchronized Shocks

Unsynchronized high-energy shocks are recommended

- For a patient who is pulseless
- For a patient demonstrating clinical deterioration (in prearrest), such as those with severe shock or polymorphic VT, when you think a delay in converting the rhythm will result in pulseless arrest
- When you are unsure whether monomorphic or polymorphic VT is present in the unstable patient

Should the unsynchronized shock cause VF (occurring in only a very small minority of patients despite the theoretical risk), immediately attempt defibrillation.

Energy Doses for Cardioversion

Select the energy dose for the specific type of rhythm. For cardioversion of atrial fibrillation, the recommended initial monophasic energy dose is 100 J to 200 J with a monophasic waveform. A dose of 100 J to 120 J is reasonable with a biphasic waveform. Escalate the second and subsequent shock dose as needed.

Cardioversion of atrial flutter and SVT generally requires less energy. An initial energy dose of 50 J to 100 J monophasic damped sinusoidal (MDS) waveform is often sufficient. If the initial 50-J dose fails, increase the dose in a stepwise fashion.

Cardioversion with a biphasic waveform is available, but more data is needed before detailed comparative dosing recommendations can be made.

Synchronized Cardioversion Technique

Introduction

Synchronized cardioversion is the treatment of choice when a patient has a symptomatic (unstable) reentry SVT or VT with pulses. It is also recommended to treat unstable atrial fibrillation and unstable atrial flutter.

Cardioversion is unlikely to be effective for treatment of junctional tachycardia or ectopic or multifocal atrial tachycardia because these rhythms have an automatic focus arising from cells that are spontaneously depolarizing at a rapid rate. Delivery of a shock generally cannot stop these rhythms and may actually increase the rate of the tachyarrhythmia.

In synchronized cardioversion shocks are administered through adhesive electrodes or handheld paddles. *You will need to place the defibrillator/monitor in synchronized (sync) mode.* The sync mode is designed to deliver energy just after the R wave of the QRS complex.

Technique

Follow these steps to perform synchronized cardioversion. Modify for your specific device.

Step	Action
1	Sedate all conscious patients unless unstable or deteriorating rapidly
2	Turn on the defibrillator (monophasic or biphasic).
3	Attach monitor leads to the patient ("white to right, red to ribs, what's left over to the left shoulder") and ensure proper display of the patient's rhythm. Position adhesive electrode (conductor) pads on the patient.
4	Press the SYNC control button to engage synchronization mode.
5	Look for markers on the R wave indicating sync mode.
6	Adjust monitor gain if necessary until sync markers occur with each R wave.
7	Select the appropriate energy level. Deliver monophasic synchronized shocks in the following sequence: table below *Biphasic waveforms using lower energy are acceptable if documented to be clinically equivalent or superior to reports of monophasic shock success. Extrapolation from elective cardioversion of atrial fibrillation supports an initial biphasic dose of 100 J to 120 J with escalation as needed. Consult the device manufacturer for specific recommendations.
8	Announce to team members: "Charging defibrillator—stand clear!"
9	Press the CHARGE button.
10	Clear the patient when the defibrillator is charged. (See Foundation Facts: Clearing for Defibrillation, in the VF/Pulseless VT Case.)
11	Press the SHOCK button(s).
12	Check the monitor. If tachycardia persists, increase the energy level (joules) according to the electrical cardioversion algorithm.
13	Activate the sync mode after delivery of each synchronized shock. *Most defibrillators default back to the unsynchronized mode after delivery of a synchronized shock. This default allows an immediate shock if cardioversion produces VF.*

If	Sequence*
Atrial fibrillation	100 to 200 J, 300 J, 360 J
Stable monomorphic VT	100 J, 200 J, 300 J, 360 J
Other SVT Atrial flutter	50 J, 100 J, 200 J, 300 J, 360 J
Polymorphic VT (irregular form and rate) and unstable	Treat as VF with high-energy shock (defibrillation doses)

Stable Tachycardia Case

Introduction

This case reviews assessment and management of a *stable patient with a rapid heart rate.* Patients with heart rates exceeding 100 bpm have a tachyarrhythmia or tachycardia. In this case we will use the terms *tachycardia* and *tachyarrhythmia* interchangeably. Note that sinus tachycardia is excluded from the treatment algorithm. Sinus tachycardia is almost always physiologic, developing in response to a compromise in stroke volume or a condition that requires an increase in cardiac output (eg, fever, hypovolemia). Treatment involves identification and correction of that underlying problem.

You must be able to classify the type of tachycardia (wide or narrow; regular or irregular) and implement appropriate interventions as outlined in the ACLS Tachycardia Algorithm. During this case you will

- Perform initial assessment and management
- Treat regular narrow-complex rhythms (except sinus tachycardia) with vagal maneuvers and adenosine

If the rhythm does not convert, you will monitor the patient and transport or obtain expert consultation. If the patient becomes clinically unstable, you will prepare for immediate unsynchronized shock or synchronized cardioversion as discussed in the Unstable Tachycardia Case.

Learning Objectives

At the end of this case, you should be able to demonstrate

1. How to perform an initial patient assessment that can identify symptoms due to a stable tachycardia
2. How to identify sinus tachycardia and understand that treatment involves identification of an underlying cause
3. How to identify tachycardias with narrow or wide QRS complexes
4. How to treat stable tachycardias according to the ACLS Tachycardia Algorithm
5. When to consider expert consultation

Rhythms for Stable Tachycardia

Tachycardias can be classified in several ways based on the appearance of the QRS complex and whether they are regular or irregular:

- Narrow–QRS-complex (SVT) tachycardias (QRS <0.12 second)
  - Sinus tachycardia
  - Atrial fibrillation
  - Atrial flutter
  - AV nodal reentry

- Wide–QRS-complex tachycardias (QRS ≥0.12 second)
  - Monomorphic VT
  - Polymorphic VT

- Regular or irregular tachycardias
  - Irregular narrow-complex tachycardias are probably atrial fibrillation

Drugs for Stable Tachycardia	This case involves the following drug:

- Adenosine

Several agents are also used to provide analgesia and sedation during electrical cardioversion. These agents are not covered in the ACLS Provider Course.

Approach to Stable Tachycardia

Introduction	In this case a stable tachycardia refers to a condition in which the patient has

- Heart rate >100 bpm
- No significant signs or symptoms caused by the increased rate
- An underlying cardiac electrical abnormality that generates the rhythm

Questions to Determine Classification	Classification of the tachycardia depends on the careful clinical evaluation of these questions:

- Are symptoms present or absent?
- Are symptoms due to the tachycardia?
- Is the patient stable or unstable?
- Is the QRS complex narrow or wide?
- Is the rhythm regular or irregular?
- Is the rhythm sinus tachycardia?

The answers guide subsequent diagnosis and treatment.

Foundation Facts: **Understanding Sinus Tachycardia**	Sinus tachycardia is a heart rate that is greater than 100 bpm and is generated by sinus node discharge. The heart rate in sinus tachycardia does not exceed 180 bpm except in young people during strenuous physical exercise. At rest sinus tachycardia usually does not exceed 120 to 130 bpm, and it has a gradual onset and gradual termination. Reentry SVT has an abrupt onset and termination.

Sinus tachycardia is caused by *external influences* on the heart, such as fever, blood loss, or exercise. These are systemic conditions, not cardiac conditions. Sinus tachycardia is a regular rhythm, although the rate may be slowed by vagal maneuvers. Cardioversion is contraindicated.

β-Blockers may cause clinical deterioration if the cardiac output falls when a *compensatory* tachycardia is blocked. This is because cardiac output is determined by the volume of blood ejected by the ventricles with each contraction (stroke volume) and the heart rate.

Cardiac Output (CO) = Stroke Volume (SV) × Heart Rate

If a condition such as a large AMI limits ventricular function (severe heart failure or cardiogenic shock), the heart compensates by increasing the heart rate. If you attempt to reduce the heart rate in patients with a compensatory tachycardia, cardiac output will fall and the patient's condition will likely deteriorate.

In sinus tachycardia the goal is to identify and treat the underlying systemic cause.

Managing Stable Tachycardia: the ACLS Tachycardia Algorithm

Introduction

As noted in the Unstable Tachycardia Case, the key to management of a patient with any tachycardia is to determine whether pulses are present, and if pulses are present to determine whether the patient is stable or unstable and then to provide treatment based on patient condition and rhythm. If the patient is pulseless, manage the patient according to the ACLS Pulseless Arrest Algorithm. If the patient has pulses, manage the patient according to the ACLS Tachycardia Algorithm.

The ACLS Provider Course focuses on the initial parts of the ACLS Tachycardia Algorithm (those boxes that are screened in the Guidelines and the ECC Handbook). These screened boxes (ie, the text in the boxes appears lighter than regular text) include actions that are intended for in-hospital use or when expert consultation is available.

Overview

If a tachycardia and a pulse are present, perform assessment and management steps guided by the BLS Primary Survey and the ACLS Secondary Survey. Determine if significant symptoms or signs are present and if these symptoms and signs are due to the tachycardia. This will direct you to either the *stable* or *unstable* branch of the algorithm.

If significant signs or symptoms are due to the tachycardia, then the tachycardia is *unstable* and immediate cardioversion is indicated (see the Unstable Tachycardia Case). If the patient develops *pulseless VT,* deliver unsynchronized high-energy shocks (defibrillation energy) and follow the ACLS Pulseless Arrest Algorithm. If the patient has *polymorphic VT and is unstable,* treat the rhythm as VF and deliver high-energy unsynchronized shocks (ie, defibrillation energy).

In this case the patient is *stable,* and you will manage according to the stable (left side) of the ACLS Tachycardia Algorithm (Figure 17). A precise identification of the rhythm (eg, reentry SVT, atrial flutter) may not be possible at this time.

Application of the ACLS Tachycardia Algorithm for the Stable Patient

Introduction

In this case a *patient has stable tachycardia with a pulse.* Conduct the steps outlined in the ACLS Tachycardia Algorithm to evaluate and manage the patient.

Primary and Secondary Surveys (Box 2)

Using the BLS Primary Survey and the ACLS Secondary Survey to guide your approach, evaluate the patient and do the following as necessary:

- Support the airway, breathing, and circulation.
- Give oxygen; monitor oxygen saturation.
- Obtain an ECG to identify the rhythm; check blood pressure.
- Identify and treat reversible causes.

If symptoms persist, proceed to Box 3.

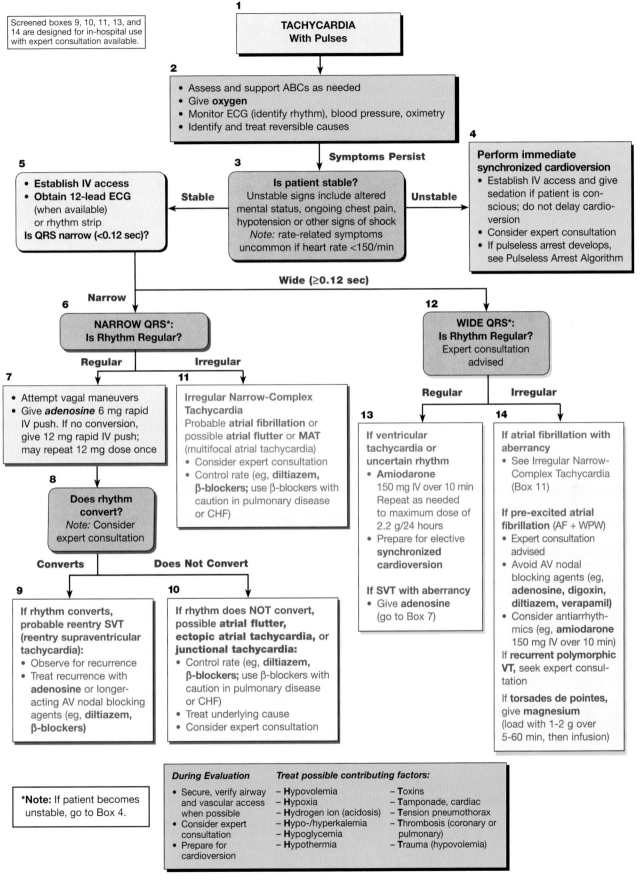

Figure 17. ACLS Tachycardia Algorithm.

Decision Point: Stable or Unstable (Box 3)

Unstable

If the patient is *unstable* with signs or symptoms as a result of the tachycardia (eg, altered mental status, ongoing chest pain, hypotension, or other signs of shock), go to Box 4 (perform immediate synchronized cardioversion). See the Unstable Tachycardia Case.

Stable

If the patient is stable, go to Box 5.

IV Access 12-Lead ECG (Box 5)

If the patient with tachycardia is *stable* (ie, no serious signs or symptoms related to the tachycardia), you have time to evaluate the rhythm and decide on treatment options. Establish IV access if not already obtained. Obtain a 12-lead ECG (when available) or rhythm strip to determine if the QRS is narrow or wide.

Decision Point: Narrow or Wide (Box 6, Box 12)

The path of treatment is now determined by whether the QRS is narrow or wide and whether the rhythm is regular or irregular. If a wide-complex rhythm is present and the patient is stable, expert consultation is advised.

Identify QRS	If the rhythm is	Go to
Narrow QRS (Box 6)	Regular rhythm	Box 7
	Irregular rhythm	Box 11*
Wide QRS (Box 12)	Regular rhythm	Box 13*
	Irregular rhythm	Box 14*

*Expert consultation is advised.

Foundation Facts: **Treating Tachycardia**	You may not always be able to distinguish between supraventricular (aberrant) and ventricular wide-complex rhythms. If you are unsure, be aware that most wide-complex (broad-complex) tachycardias are *ventricular* in origin. If a patient is *pulseless* or with severe signs of decompensating *shock*, follow the ACLS Pulseless Arrest Algorithm. If a patient becomes *unstable*, do not delay treatment for further rhythm analysis. For *stable* patients with wide-complex tachycardias, transport and monitor, or consult an expert because treatment has the potential for harm.

Narrow QRS, Regular Rhythm (Box 7)

Identify QRS	If the rhythm is	Go to
Narrow QRS	Regular rhythm	Box 7

The therapy for narrow QRS with regular rhythm is

- Attempt vagal maneuvers
- Give adenosine

Vagal maneuvers and adenosine are the preferred initial interventions for terminating narrow-complex tachycardias that are symptomatic and supraventricular in origin (SVT). Vagal maneuvers alone (Valsalva maneuver or carotid sinus massage) will terminate about 20% to 25% of SVT. Adenosine is required for the remainder.

If SVT does not respond to vagal maneuvers:

- Give **adenosine** 6 mg as a rapid IV push.
- If SVT does not convert within 1 to 2 minutes, give a second dose of adenosine: 12 mg rapid IV push.
- If SVT does not convert within 1 to 2 minutes, give a third dose of adenosine: 12 mg rapid IV push.

For IV administration, give adenosine in a large (eg, antecubital) vein over 1 second. Follow with a 20-mL saline flush and elevate the arm immediately.

Adenosine increases AV block and will terminate approximately 90% of reentry arrhythmias within 2 minutes. Adenosine will not terminate atrial flutter or atrial fibrillation but will slow AV conduction, allowing for identification of flutter or fibrillation waves. Adenosine is contraindicated in wide-complex tachycardias unless they are known to *definitely* be reentrant in origin (usually by prior history or ECG).

Adenosine is safe and effective in pregnancy. Adenosine does, however, have several important drug interactions. Larger doses may be required for patients with significant blood levels of theophylline, caffeine, or theobromide. The initial dose should be reduced to 3 mg in patients taking dipyrimadole or carbamazepine. There have been recent case reports of prolonged asystole following adenosine administration to patients with transplanted hearts or following central venous administration, so lower doses such as 3 mg may be considered in these situations.

Adenosine may cause bronchospasm; avoid using it in patients with reactive airway disease.

Does the Rhythm Convert? (Box 8)

Narrow QRS	Regular Rhythm
Does the rhythm convert with adenosine? (Box 8)	

YES

If the rhythm converts, it is probable reentry SVT. Observe for recurrence. Treat recurrence with adenosine or longer-acting AV nodal blocking agents (eg, diltiazem, β-blockers). Typically you should obtain expert consultation if the tachycardia recurs.

NO

If the rhythm does not convert, it is possible atrial flutter, ectopic atrial tachycardia, or junctional tachycardia. Obtain expert consultation about diagnosis and treatment.

Wide- (Broad-) Complex Tachycardias (Box 12)

Identify QRS	If the rhythm is	Go to
Wide QRS (Box 12)	Regular rhythm	Box 13
	Irregular rhythm	Box 14

Wide-complex tachycardias are defined as having a QRS of 0.12 second or greater. *Expert consultation is advised. It is not a consideration or an option.*

The most common forms of life-threatening wide-complex tachycardias likely to deteriorate to VF are

- Monomorphic VT
- Polymorphic VT

Determine if the rhythm is regular or irregular (Box 12). A regular wide-complex tachycardia is presumed to be VT until proven otherwise. An irregular wide-complex tachycardia may be atrial fibrillation with aberrancy, pre-excited atrial fibrillation (ie, atrial fibrillation with Wolff-Parkinson-White syndrome). These are advanced rhythms requiring additional expertise or expert consultation.

Therapy for Regular Wide-Complex Tachycardias (Box 13)

Identify QRS	If the rhythm is	Go to
Wide QRS	Regular rhythm	Box 13

Providers should consider the need to seek expert consultation when treating wide-complex tachycardias.

Synchronized cardioversion is appropriate for treating wide-complex tachycardia of unknown type. You should prepare for synchronized cardioversion as soon as a wide-complex tachycardia is detected.

If the rhythm is likely VT in a stable patient, IV antiarrhythmic drugs may be effective. We recommend amiodarone 150 mg IV over 10 minutes. Repeat once if rhythm persists, while obtaining expert consultation.

ACLS Tachycardia Algorithm: Advanced Management Steps

Some ACLS providers may be familiar with the differential diagnosis and therapy of stable tachycardias that do not respond to initial treatment. The basic ACLS provider is expected to recognize a stable narrow-complex or wide-complex tachycardia and classify the rhythm as regular or irregular. Regular narrow-complex tachycardias may be treated initially with vagal maneuvers and adenosine. If these are unsuccessful, the ACLS provider should transport or *seek expert consultation*.

If ACLS providers have experience with the differential diagnosis and therapy of stable tachycardias beyond initial management, the ACLS Tachycardia Algorithm lists additional steps and pharmacologic agents used in the treatment of these arrhythmias, both for rate control and termination of the arrhythmia.

> **If at any point you become uncertain or uncomfortable during the treatment of a stable patient, seek expert consultation. The treatment of stable patients may await expert consultation because treatment has the potential for harm.**

Acute Stroke Case

Introduction

The identification and initial management of patients with acute stroke is within the scope of an ACLS provider. This case covers *principles of out-of-hospital care* and *fundamental aspects of initial in-hospital acute stroke care.*

Out-of-hospital acute stroke care focuses on

- Rapid identification and assessment of patients with stroke
- Rapid transport (with prearrival notification) to a facility capable of providing acute stroke care

In-hospital acute stroke care includes the

- Ability to rapidly determine patient eligibility for fibrinolytic therapy
- Administration of fibrinolytic therapy to appropriate candidates, with availability of neurologic medical supervision within target times
- Initiation of the stroke pathway and patient admission to a stroke unit if available

The target times and goals are recommended by the National Institute of Neurological Disorders and Stroke (NINDS). NINDS has recommended measurable goals for the evaluation of stroke patients. These targets or goals should be achieved for at least 80% of patients with acute stroke.

Learning Objectives

By the end of this case you should be able to

1. Describe the major signs and symptoms of stroke
2. Classify stroke and explain stroke type-specific treatments
3. Recognize signs and symptoms of stroke and recall their differential diagnoses
4. Demonstrate the use of 1 of the 2 out-of-hospital stroke scales (screening tools) to identify patients with suspected stroke
5. Apply the 7 D's of stroke care and explain why timely action is crucial
6. Follow the ACLS Suspected Stroke Algorithm, including NINDS time goals
7. Recall that rapid transport to a healthcare facility capable of providing acute stroke care is recommended when stroke is suspected
8. Recall general eligibility criteria for fibrinolytic therapy and activation of the stroke team

Potential Arrhythmias With Stroke

The ECG does not take priority over obtaining a CT scan. No arrhythmias are specific for stroke, but the ECG may identify evidence of a recent AMI or arrhythmias such as atrial fibrillation as a cause of an embolic stroke. Many patients with stroke may demonstrate arrhythmias. But if the patient is hemodynamically stable, most arrhythmias will not require treatment.

Drugs for Stroke

This case involves these drugs:

- Approved fibrinolytic agent (tissue plasminogen activator [tPA])
- Glucose (D_{50})
- Labetalol
- Nitroprusside
- Nicardipine
- Aspirin

See the pharmacology module on the student CD or the ECC Handbook for more information.

Foundation Facts:

Major Types of Stroke

Stroke is a general term. It refers to acute neurologic impairment that follows interruption in blood supply to a specific area of the brain. Although expeditious stroke care is important to all patients, this case emphasizes reperfusion therapy for acute ischemic stroke.

The major types of stroke are

- Ischemic stroke—accounts for 85% of all strokes and is usually caused by an occlusion of an artery to a region of the brain
- Hemorrhagic stroke—accounts for 15% of all strokes and occurs when a blood vessel in the brain suddenly ruptures into the surrounding tissue. Fibrinolytics are contraindicated in this type of stroke. Avoid anticoagulants.

Approach to Stroke Care

Introduction

Each year in the United States about 700,000 people suffer a new or repeated stroke. About 1 in 15 deaths in the United States is due to stroke.

Early recognition of acute ischemic stroke is important because IV fibrinolytic treatment must be provided within 3 hours of onset of symptoms. Most strokes occur at home, and only half of acute stroke patients use EMS for transport to the hospital. Stroke patients often deny or try to rationalize their symptoms. Even high-risk patients, such as those with atrial fibrillation or hypertension, fail to recognize the signs of stroke. This delays activation of EMS and treatment, resulting in increased morbidity and mortality.

Community and professional education is essential, and it has been successful in increasing the proportion of eligible stroke victims treated with fibrinolytics. Healthcare providers, hospitals, and communities must continue to develop systems to improve the efficiency and effectiveness of stroke care.

Foundation Facts:

Stroke Chain of Survival

The goal of stroke care is to minimize brain injury and maximize the patient's recovery. The Stroke Chain of Survival (Figure 18) described by the AHA and the American Stroke Association is similar to the Chain of Survival for sudden cardiac arrest. It links actions to be taken by patients, family members, and healthcare providers to maximize stroke recovery. These links are

- Rapid recognition and reaction to stroke warning signs
- Rapid EMS dispatch
- Rapid EMS system transport and prearrival notification to the receiving hospital
- Rapid diagnosis and treatment in the hospital

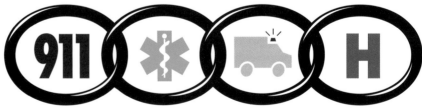

Figure 18. Stroke Chain of Survival.

Foundation Facts:

The 7 D's of Stroke Care

The 7 D's of stroke care highlight the major steps in diagnosis and treatment of stroke and key points at which delays can occur:

- **Detection** of the onset of signs and symptoms of stroke
- **Dispatch** of EMS (by telephoning 911 or the emergency response number)
- **Delivery** with advanced prehospital notification to a hospital capable of providing acute stroke care
- **Door** of the ED, including arrival and urgent triage in the ED
- **Data**, including computed tomography (CT) scan and interpretation of the scan
- **Decision** regarding treatment, including fibrinolytics
- **Drug** administration (as appropriate) and postadministration monitoring

For more information on these critical elements, see the ACLS Suspected Stroke Algorithm (Figure 19).

Goals of Stroke Care

The ACLS Suspected Stroke Algorithm (Figure 19) emphasizes important elements of out-of-hospital care for possible stroke patients. These actions include a stroke scale or screen and rapid transport to the hospital. As with ACS, prior notification of the receiving hospital speeds the care of the stroke patient upon arrival.

Critical in-hospital time goals have been established by NINDS for assessment and management of patients with suspected stroke. This algorithm reviews the critical in-hospital time periods for patient assessment and treatment:

1. Immediate general assessment by the stroke team, emergency physician, or another expert within *10 minutes* of arrival; order urgent noncontrast CT scan
2. Neurologic assessment by the stroke team or their designee and CT scan performed within *25 minutes* of hospital arrival
3. Interpretation of the CT scan within *45 minutes* of ED arrival
4. Initiation of fibrinolytic therapy in appropriate patients (those without contraindications) within 1 hour of hospital arrival and 3 hours from symptom onset
5. Door-to-admission time of 3 hours

Foundation

Facts:

NINDS

The National Institute of Neurological Disorders and Stroke (NINDS) is a branch of the National Institutes of Health (NIH). The mission of NINDS is to reduce the burden of neurologic disease by supporting and conducting research. NINDS researchers have studied stroke and reviewed data leading to recommendations for acute stroke care. NINDS has set critical time goals for assessment and management of stroke victims based on experience obtained in large studies of stroke victims.

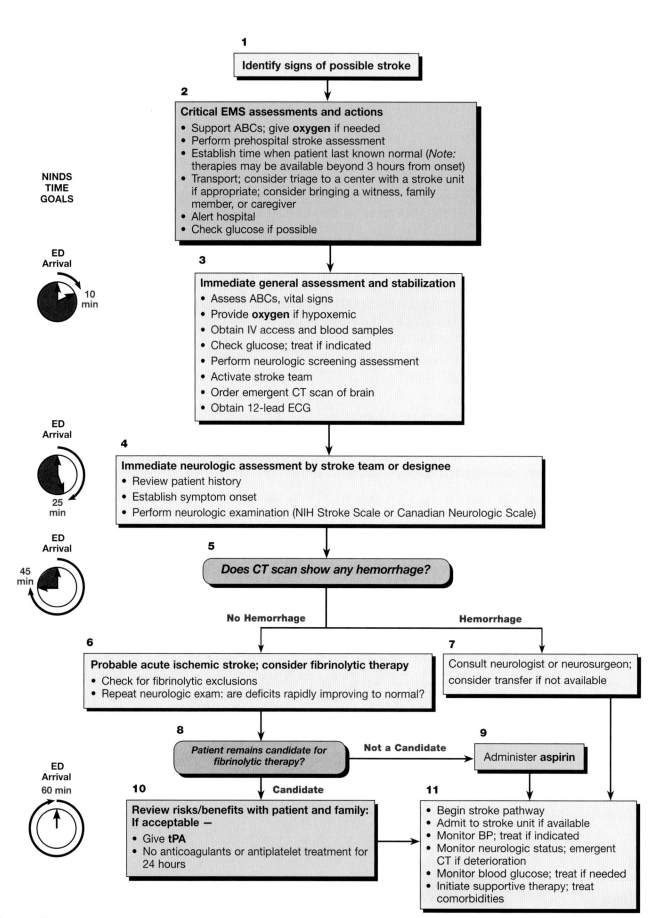

1
Identify signs of possible stroke

2
Critical EMS assessments and actions
- Support ABCs; give **oxygen** if needed
- Perform prehospital stroke assessment
- Establish time when patient last known normal (*Note:* therapies may be available beyond 3 hours from onset)
- Transport; consider triage to a center with a stroke unit if appropriate; consider bringing a witness, family member, or caregiver
- Alert hospital
- Check glucose if possible

NINDS
TIME
GOALS

ED
Arrival

10 min

3
Immediate general assessment and stabilization
- Assess ABCs, vital signs
- Provide **oxygen** if hypoxemic
- Obtain IV access and blood samples
- Check glucose; treat if indicated
- Perform neurologic screening assessment
- Activate stroke team
- Order emergent CT scan of brain
- Obtain 12-lead ECG

ED
Arrival

25 min

4
Immediate neurologic assessment by stroke team or designee
- Review patient history
- Establish symptom onset
- Perform neurologic examination (NIH Stroke Scale or Canadian Neurologic Scale)

ED
Arrival

45 min

5
Does CT scan show any hemorrhage?

No Hemorrhage | Hemorrhage

6
Probable acute ischemic stroke; consider fibrinolytic therapy
- Check for fibrinolytic exclusions
- Repeat neurologic exam: are deficits rapidly improving to normal?

7
Consult neurologist or neurosurgeon; consider transfer if not available

8
Patient remains candidate for fibrinolytic therapy?

Not a Candidate

9
Administer **aspirin**

ED
Arrival
60 min

10
Review risks/benefits with patient and family: If acceptable —
- Give **tPA**
- No anticoagulants or antiplatelet treatment for 24 hours

Candidate

11
- Begin stroke pathway
- Admit to stroke unit if available
- Monitor BP; treat if indicated
- Monitor neurologic status; emergent CT if deterioration
- Monitor blood glucose; treat if needed
- Initiate supportive therapy; treat comorbidities

Figure 19. The Suspected Stroke Algorithm.

Critical Time Periods

Patients with acute ischemic stroke have a time-dependent benefit for fibrinolytic therapy similar to that of patients with ST-segment elevation MI, but this time-dependent benefit is much shorter.

The critical time period for administration of *intravenous* fibrinolytic therapy begins with the onset of symptoms. Critical time periods from hospital arrival are summarized below:

• Immediate general assessment	10 minutes
• Immediate neurologic assessment	25 minutes
• Acquisition of head CT	25 minutes
• Interpretation of the CT Scan	45 minutes
• Administration of fibrinolytics, timed from ED arrival	60 minutes
• Administration of fibrinolytics, timed from onset of symptoms	3 hours
• Admission to a monitored bed	3 hours

Application of the Algorithm for Suspected Stroke

We will now discuss the steps in the algorithm, as well as other related topics:

- Identification of signs of possible stroke (Box 1)
- Critical EMS assessments and actions (Box 2)
- Immediate general assessment and stabilization (Box 3)
- Immediate neurologic assessment by the stroke team or designee (Box 4)
- CT scan: hemorrhage or no hemorrhage (Box 5)
- Fibrinolytic therapy risk stratification if candidate
- General stroke care (Box 11)

Identification of Signs of Possible Stroke (Box 1)

Warning Signs and Symptoms

The signs and symptoms of a stroke may be subtle. They include

- Sudden weakness or numbness of the face, arm, or leg, especially on one side of the body
- Sudden confusion
- Trouble speaking or understanding
- Sudden trouble seeing in one or both eyes
- Sudden trouble walking
- Dizziness or loss of balance or coordination
- Sudden severe headache with no known cause

Activate EMS System Immediately

Stroke patients and their families must be educated to activate the EMS system (usually by phoning 911) as soon as they detect potential signs or symptoms of stroke. Currently half of all stroke patients are driven to the ED by family or friends.

The EMS system provides the safest and most efficient method of emergency transport to the hospital. Advantages include the following:

- EMS personnel can identify and transport to a hospital capable of providing acute stroke care and notify the hospital of the patient's impending arrival.
- Prearrival notification allows the hospital to prepare to evaluate and manage the patient efficiently.

Emergency medical dispatchers also play a critical role in timely treatment of potential stroke. They

- Identify possible patients with stroke
- Provide high-priority dispatch
- Instruct bystanders in lifesaving CPR skills or other supportive care if needed, while EMS providers are on the way.

Stroke Assessment Tools

The *2005 AHA Guidelines for CPR and ECC* recommends that all paramedics and EMT-basics be trained to recognize stroke using a validated, abbreviated out-of-hospital neurologic evaluation tool such as the

- Cincinnati Prehospital Stroke Scale (Table 5)
- Los Angeles Prehospital Stroke Screen (Table 6).

Cincinnati Prehospital Stroke Scale (CPSS)

The CPSS identifies stroke on the basis of 3 physical findings:

- Facial droop (have the patient smile or try to show teeth)
- Arm weakness (have the patient close eyes and hold both arms out)
- Abnormal speech (have the patient say, "You can't teach an old dog new tricks")

Using the CPSS, medical personnel can evaluate the patient in less than 1 minute. The presence of 1 finding on the CPSS indicates a 72% probability of stroke. The presence of all 3 findings indicates that the probability of stroke is greater than 85%.

Table 5. The Cincinnati Prehospital Stroke Scale

Test	Findings
Facial Droop: Have the patient show teeth or smile (Figure 20)	❏ **Normal**—both sides of face move equally ❏ **Abnormal**—one side of face does not move as well as the other side
Arm Drift: Patient closes eyes and extends both arms straight out, with palms up, for 10 seconds (Figure 21)	❏ **Normal**—both arms move the same or both arms do not move at all (other findings, such as pronator drift, may be helpful) ❏ **Abnormal**—one arm does not move or one arm drifts down compared with the other
Abnormal Speech: Have the patient say "you can't teach an old dog new tricks"	❏ **Normal**—patient uses correct words with no slurring ❏ **Abnormal**—patient slurs words, uses the wrong words, or is unable to speak

Kothari R, Hall K, Brott T, Broderick J. Early stroke recognition: developing an out-of-hospital NIH Stroke Scale. *Acad Emerg Med.* 1997;4:986-990.

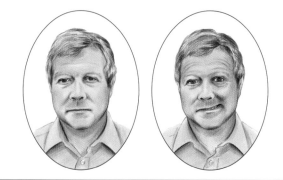

Figure 20. Facial droop.

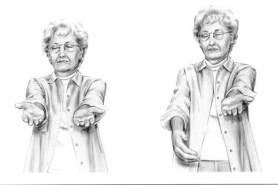

Figure 21. One-sided motor weakness (right arm).

Los Angeles Prehospital Stroke Screen (LAPSS)

The LAPSS is a more detailed screen for acute stroke. This screen builds on the physical findings of the CPSS, adding criteria for age, lack of history of seizures, symptom duration, blood glucose levels, and lack of preexisting ambulation problems. A person with positive findings on all 6 criteria has a 97% probability of an acute stroke.

Table 6. Los Angeles Prehospital Stroke Screen

For *evaluation of acute, noncomatose, nontraumatic neurologic complaint.* If items 1 through 6 are **all** checked **"Yes"** (or "Unknown"), provide prearrival notification to hospital of potential stroke patient. If any item is checked "No," return to appropriate treatment protocol. *Interpretation:* 93% of patients with stroke will have a positive LAPSS score (sensitivity = 93%), and 97% of those with a positive LAPSS score will have a stroke (specificity = 97%). Note that the patient may still be experiencing a stroke if LAPSS criteria are not met.

Criteria	Yes	Unknown	No
1. Age >45 years	❏	❏	❏
2. History of seizures or epilepsy **absent**	❏	❏	❏
3. Symptom duration <24 hours	❏	❏	❏
4. At baseline, patient is **not** wheelchair bound or bedridden	❏	❏	❏
5. Blood glucose between 60 and 400	❏	❏	❏
6. *Obvious asymmetry* (right vs left) in *any* of the following 3 exam categories **(must be unilateral):**	❏	❏	❏

	Equal	R Weak	L Weak
Facial smile/grimace	❏	❏ Droop	❏ Droop
Grip	❏	❏ Weak grip ❏ No grip	❏ Weak grip ❏ No grip
Arm strength	❏	❏ Drifts down ❏ Falls rapidly	❏ Drifts down ❏ Falls rapidly

Kidwell CS, Saver JL, Schubert GB, Eckstein M, Starkman S. Design and retrospective analysis of the Los Angeles prehospital stroke screen (LAPSS). *Prehosp Emerg Care.* 1998;2:267-273. Kidwell CS, Starkman S, Eckstein M, Weems K, Saver JL. Identifying stroke in the field: prospective validation of the Los Angeles Prehospital Stroke Screen (LAPSS). *Stroke.* 2000;31:71-76.

Critical EMS Assessments and Actions (Box 2)

Introduction

Prehospital EMS providers must minimize the interval between the onset of symptoms and patient arrival in the ED. Specific stroke therapy can be provided only in the appropriate receiving hospital ED, so time in the field only delays (and may prevent) definitive therapy. More extensive assessments and initiation of supportive therapies can continue en route to the hospital or in the ED.

EMS Assessments and Actions (Box 2)

To provide the best outcome for the patient with potential stroke:

Identify signs	Define and recognize the signs of stroke.
Support ABCs	Support the ABCs and give oxygen if needed.
Do stroke assessment	Perform a rapid out-of-hospital stroke assessment (CPSS or LAPSS).
Establish time	Determine when the patient was last known to be normal or at neurologic baseline. This represents time zero. If the patient wakes from sleep with symptoms of stroke, time zero is the last time the patient was seen to be normal.
Transport	Transport the patient rapidly and consider triage to a stroke center. During transport support cardiopulmonary function. If possible, bring a witness, family member, or caregiver with the patient to confirm time of onset of stroke symptoms.
Alert hospital	Provide prearrival notification to the receiving hospital.
Assess neurologic status	Identify neurologic deficits and monitor neurologic status during transport.
Check glucose	During transport, check blood glucose if protocols or medical control allows.

The patient with acute stroke is at risk for respiratory compromise from aspiration, upper airway obstruction, and hypoventilation. Neurogenic pulmonary edema is a rare complication. Hypoxemia will exacerbate and extend ischemic brain injury, and it has been associated with worse outcome from stroke.

Both out-of-hospital and in-hospital medical personnel should provide supplementary oxygen to hypoxemic (ie, oxygen saturation <92%) stroke patients or patients for whom oxygen saturation is unknown.

Foundation Facts:

Stroke Centers and Stroke Units

Initial evidence indicates a favorable benefit from triage of stroke patients directly to designated stroke centers, but the concept of routine out-of-hospital triage of stroke patients requires continued evaluation.

Each receiving hospital should define its capability for treating patients with acute stroke and should communicate this information to the EMS system and the community. Although not every hospital has the resources to safely administer fibrinolytics, every hospital with an ED should have a written plan that describes how patients with acute stroke will be managed in that institution. The plan should

- Detail the roles of healthcare providers in the care of patients with acute stroke, including identifying sources of neurologic expertise
- Define which patients to treat with fibrinolytics at that facility
- Describe when patient transfer to another hospital with a dedicated stroke unit is appropriate

When a stroke unit with a multidisciplinary team experienced in managing stroke is available within a reasonable transport interval, patients with stroke who require hospitalization should be admitted to a stroke unit.

Studies have documented improvement in 1-year survival rate, functional outcomes, and quality of life when patients hospitalized for acute stroke receive care in a dedicated unit with a specialized team.

Immediate General Assessment and Stabilization (Box 3)

Introduction

Once the patient arrives in the ED, a number of assessment and management activities must occur quickly. Protocols should be used to minimize delay in definitive diagnosis and therapy.

> **The goal of the stroke team, emergency physician, or another expert should be to assess the patient with suspected stroke within *10 minutes of arrival* in the ED (Box 3).**

Initial ED Assessment and Stabilization

ED providers should do the following:

Step	Actions
Assess ABCs	Assess the ABCs and evaluate baseline vital signs.
Provide oxygen	Provide oxygen if the patient is hypoxemic (<92% saturation). Consider oxygen administration if the patient is not hypoxemic.
Establish IV access and obtain blood samples	Establish IV access and obtain blood samples for baseline blood count, coagulation studies, and blood glucose. Do not let this delay obtaining a CT scan of the brain.
Check glucose	Promptly treat hypoglycemia.
Perform neurologic assessment	Perform a neurologic screening assessment. Use the National Institute of Health (NIH) Stroke Scale, Canadian Neurological Scale, or similar tool.

(continued)

Step	Actions
Activate the stroke team	Activate the stroke team or arrange consultation with a stroke expert based on predetermined protocols.
Order CT brain scan	Order an emergent CT scan of the brain. Have it read promptly by a qualified physician.
Obtain 12-lead ECG	Obtain a 12-lead ECG, which may identify a recent or ongoing AMI or arrhythmias (eg, atrial fibrillation) as a cause of embolic stroke. A small percentage of patients with acute stroke or TIA have coexisting myocardial ischemia or other abnormalities.
	Life-threatening arrhythmias can follow or accompany stroke, particularly intracerebral hemorrhage. If the patient is hemodynamically stable, treatment of non–life-threatening arrhythmias (bradycardia, VT, and AV conduction blocks) may not be necessary.
	Do not delay the CT scan to obtain the ECG.

Immediate Neurologic Assessment by Stroke Team (Box 4)

Overview

The stroke team, neurovascular consultant, or emergency physician does the following:

- Reviews the patient's history, performs a general physical examination, and establishes time of symptom onset
- Performs a neurologic examination

The goal for neurologic assessment is within *25 minutes of patient's arrival* in the ED (Box 4).

Establish Symptom Onset

Establishing the time of symptom onset may require interviewing out-of-hospital providers, witnesses, and family members to determine the time the patient was last known to be normal.

Neurologic Examination

Assess the patient's neurologic status using one of the following:

- National Institutes of Health Stroke Scale
- Canadian Neurological Scale

National Institutes of Health Stroke Scale (NIHSS)
The NIHSS involves 15 items used to assess the responsive stroke patient. This is a validated measure of stroke severity based on a detailed neurologic examination. A detailed discussion is beyond the scope of the ACLS Provider Course.

Canadian Neurological Scale (CNS)
The CNS assesses the neurologic function of a responsive stroke patient. It includes assessment of level of consciousness (LOC), orientation, aphasia, and motor strength. A detailed discussion is beyond the scope of the ACLS Provider Course.

CT Scan: Hemorrhage or No Hemorrhage (Box 5)

Introduction

A critical decision point in the assessment of the patient with acute stroke is the performance and interpretation of a noncontrast CT scan to differentiate ischemic from hemorrhagic stroke. Assessment also includes identifying other structural abnormalities that may be responsible for the patient's symptoms or that represent contraindication to fibrinolytic therapy. The initial noncontrast CT scan is the most important test for an acute stroke patient.

- If a CT scan is not readily available, stabilize the patient and promptly transfer to a facility with this capability.
- Do not give aspirin, heparin, or tPA until the CT scan has ruled out intracranial hemorrhage.

> The CT scan should be **completed within 25 minutes** of the patient's arrival in the ED and should be **read within 45 minutes from performance** (Box 5).

Decision Point: Hemorrhage or No Hemorrhage

Emergent CT or magnetic resonance imaging (MRI) scans of patients with suspected stroke should be promptly interpreted by a physician skilled in neuroimaging interpretation. The presence of hemorrhage versus no hemorrhage determines the next steps in treatment.

Yes, hemorrhage is present.
If hemorrhage is noted on the CT scan, the patient is not a candidate for fibrinolytics. Consult a neurologist or neurosurgeon. Consider transfer for appropriate care (Box 7).

No, hemorrhage is not present.
If the CT scan shows no evidence of hemorrhage and no sign of other abnormality (eg, tumor, recent stroke), the patient may be a candidate for fibrinolytic therapy.

If hemorrhage is not present on the initial CT scan and the patient is not a candidate for fibrinolytics for other reasons, consider giving aspirin (Box 9) either rectally or orally after performing a swallowing screen (see below). Although aspirin is not a time-critical intervention, it is appropriate to administer aspirin in the ED if the patient is not a candidate for fibrinolysis. The patient must be able to safely swallow before aspirin is given orally. Otherwise use the suppository form.

Admit the patient to a stroke unit (if available) for careful monitoring.

Fibrinolytic Therapy

Introduction

Several studies have shown a higher likelihood of good-to-excellent functional outcome when tPA is given to adults with acute ischemic stroke within 3 hours of onset of symptoms. But these results are obtained when tPA is given by physicians in hospitals with a stroke protocol that rigorously adheres to the eligibility criteria and therapeutic regimen of the NINDS protocol. Evidence from prospective randomized studies in adults also documents a greater likelihood of benefit the earlier treatment begins.

AHA and stroke guidelines recommend giving IV tPA to patients with acute ischemic stroke who meet the NINDS eligibility criteria if it is given by

- Physicians using a clearly defined institutional protocol
- A knowledgeable interdisciplinary team familiar with stroke care
- An institution with commitment to comprehensive stroke care and rehabilitation

The superior outcomes reported in both community and tertiary care hospitals in the NINDS trials can be difficult to replicate in hospitals with less experience in, and institutional commitment to, acute stroke care. There is strong evidence to avoid all delays and treat patients as soon as possible. Failure to adhere to protocol is associated with an increased rate of complications, particularly risk of intracranial hemorrhage.

Evaluate for Fibrinolytic Therapy

If the CT scan is negative for hemorrhage, the patient may be a candidate for fibrinolytic therapy. Immediately perform further eligibility and risk stratification:

- If the CT scan shows no hemorrhage, the probability of acute ischemic stroke remains. *Review inclusion and exclusion criteria for IV fibrinolytic therapy (Table 7) and repeat the neurologic exam* (NIH Stroke Scale or Canadian Neurological Scale).
- If the patient's neurologic function is rapidly improving toward normal, fibrinolytics may be unnecessary.

Potential Adverse Effects

As with all drugs, fibrinolytics have potential adverse effects. At this point weigh the patient's risk for adverse events against the potential benefit and discuss with the patient and family.

- Confirm that no exclusion criteria are present.
- Consider risks and benefits.
- Be prepared to monitor and treat any potential complications.

The major complication of IV tPA for stroke is intracranial hemorrhage. Other bleeding complications may occur and may range from minor to major. Angioedema and transient hypotension may occur.

Patient Is a Candidate for Fibrinolytic Therapy

If the patient remains a candidate for fibrinolytic therapy (Box 8), discuss the risks and potential benefits with the patient or family if available (Box 10). After this discussion, if the patient/family decides to proceed with fibrinolytic therapy, give the patient tPA. Begin your institution's stroke tPA protocol, often called a "pathway of care."

> *Do not administer anticoagulants or antiplatelet treatment for 24 hours after administration of tPA, typically until a follow-up CT scan at 24 hours shows no intracranial hemorrhage.*

Intra-arterial tPA

Improved outcome from use of cerebral intra-arterial tPA has been documented. For patients with acute ischemic stroke who are not candidates for standard IV fibrinolysis, consider intra-arterial fibrinolysis in centers with the resources and expertise to provide it within the first 6 hours after onset of symptoms. Intra-arterial administration of tPA is not yet approved by the FDA.

Table 7. Fibrinolytic Checklist

All boxes must be checked before tPA can be given.

Note: The following checklist includes FDA-approved indications and contraindications for tPA administration for acute ischemic stroke. A physician with expertise in acute stroke care may modify this list.

Inclusion Criteria *(all **Yes** boxes in this section must be checked):*

Yes

❑ Age 18 years or older?
❑ Clinical diagnosis of ischemic stroke with a measurable neurologic deficit?
❑ Time of symptom onset (when patient was last seen normal) well established as <180 minutes (3 hours) before treatment would begin?

Exclusion Criteria *(all **No** boxes in "Contraindications" section must be checked):*
Contraindications:

No

❑ Evidence of intracranial hemorrhage on pretreatment noncontrast head CT?
❑ Clinical presentation suggestive of subarachnoid hemorrhage even with normal CT?
❑ CT shows multilobar infarction (hypodensity greater than one third cerebral hemisphere)?
❑ History of intracranial hemorrhage?
❑ Uncontrolled hypertension: At the time treatment should begin, systolic pressure remains >185 mm Hg or diastolic pressure remains >110 mm Hg despite repeated measurements?
❑ Known arteriovenous malformation, neoplasm, or aneurysm?
❑ Witnessed seizure at stroke onset?
❑ Active internal bleeding or acute trauma (fracture)?
❑ Acute bleeding diathesis, including but not limited to
    — Platelet count <100 000/mm^3?
    — Heparin received within 48 hours, resulting in an activated partial thromboplastin time (aPTT) that is greater than upper limit of normal for laboratory?
    — Current use of anticoagulant (eg, warfarin sodium) that has produced an elevated international normalized ratio (INR) >1.7 or prothrombin time (PT) >15 seconds?*
❑ Within 3 months of intracranial or intraspinal surgery, serious head trauma, or previous stroke?
❑ Arterial puncture at a noncompressible site within past 7 days?

Relative Contraindications/Precautions:

Recent experience suggests that under some circumstances—with careful consideration and weighing of risk-to-benefit ratio—patients may receive fibrinolytic therapy despite one or more relative contraindications. Consider the pros and cons of tPA administration carefully if any of these relative contraindications is present:

• Only minor or rapidly improving stroke symptoms (clearing spontaneously)
• Within 14 days of major surgery or serious trauma
• Recent gastrointestinal or urinary tract hemorrhage (within previous 21 days)
• Recent acute myocardial infarction (within previous 3 months)
• Postmyocardial infarction pericarditis
• Abnormal blood glucose level (<50 or >400 mg/dL [<2.8 or >22.2 mmol/L])

*In patients without recent use of oral anticoagulants or heparin, treatment with tPA can be initiated before availability of coagulation study results but should be discontinued if the INR is >1.7 or the partial thromboplastin time is elevated by local laboratory standards.

General Stroke Care (Box 11)

Introduction

The general care of all patients with stroke includes the following:

• Begin stroke pathway.
• Support airway, breathing, and circulation.
• Monitor blood glucose.
• Monitor for complications of stroke and fibrinolytic therapy.
• Transfer to general intensive care if indicated.

Begin Stroke Pathway

Admit patients to a stroke unit (if available) for careful observation (Box 11), including monitoring of blood pressure and neurologic status. If neurologic status worsens, order an emergent CT scan. Determine if cerebral edema or hemorrhage is the cause; consult neurosurgery as appropriate.

Additional stroke care includes support of the airway, oxygenation, ventilation, and nutrition. Provide normal saline to maintain intravascular volume (eg, approximately 75 to 100 mL/h) if needed.

Monitor Blood Glucose

Hyperglycemia is associated with worse clinical outcome in patients with acute ischemic stroke. But there is no direct evidence that active glucose control improves clinical outcome. There is evidence that insulin treatment of hyperglycemia in other critically ill patients improves survival rates. For this reason consider giving IV or subcutaneous insulin to lower blood glucose in patients with acute ischemic stroke when the serum glucose level is greater than 10 mmol/L (or greater than about 200 mg/dL).

Monitor for Complications of Stroke and Fibrinolytic Therapy

Prophylaxis for seizures is not recommended. But treatment of acute seizures followed by administration of anticonvulsants to prevent further seizures is recommended. Monitor the patient for signs of increased intracranial pressure. Continue to control blood pressure to reduce the potential risk of bleeding.

Hypertension Management in tPA Candidates

Although management of hypertension in the stroke patient is controversial, patients who are candidates for fibrinolytic therapy should have their blood pressure controlled to lower the risk of intracerebral hemorrhage following administration of tPA. General guidelines for the management of hypertension are outlined in Table 8.

Table 8. Approach to Elevated Blood Pressure in Acute Ischemic Stroke.

Blood Pressure Level, mm Hg	Treatment
A. Not eligible for fibrinolytic therapy	
Systolic ≤220 **or** diastolic ≤120	• Observe unless other end-organ involvement (eg, aortic dissection, acute myocardial infarction, pulmonary edema, hypertensive encephalopathy) • Treat other symptoms of stroke (eg, headach, pain, agitation, nausea, vomiting) • Treat other acute complications of stroke, including hypoxia, increased intracranial pressure, seizures, or hypoglycemia
Systolic >220 **or** diastolic 121 to 140	• Labetalol 10 to 20 mg IV for 1 to 2 minutes • May repeat or double every 10 minutes (max dose 300 mg) OR • Nicardipine 5 mg/h IV infusion as initial dose; titrate to desired effect by increasing 2.5 mg/h every 5 minutes to max of 15 mg/h • Aim for a 10% to 15% reduction in blood pressure
Diastolic >140	• Nitroprusside 0.5 µg/kg per minute IV infusion as initial dose with continuous blood pressure monitoring • Aim for a 10% to 15% reduction in blood pressure

Blood Pressure Level, mm Hg	Treatment
B. Eligible for fibrinolytic therapy	
Pretreatment	
Systolic >185 **or** diastolic >110	• Labetalol 10 to 20 mg IV for 1 to 2 minutes • May repeat 1 time or nitropaste 1 to 2 inches
During/after treatment	
Monitor blood pressure	• Check blood pressure every 15 minutes for 2 hours, then every 30 minutes for 6 hours, and finally every hour for 16 hours
Diastolic >140	• Sodium nitroprusside 0.5 µg/kg per minute IV infusion as initial dose and titrate to desired blood pressure
Systolic >230 **or** diastolic 121 to 140	• Labetalol 10 mg IV for 1 to 2 minutes • May repeat or double labetalol every 10 minutes to max dose of 300 mg, or give initial labetalol dose, then start labetalol drip at 2 to 8 mg/minutes OR • Nicardipine 5 mg/h IV infusion as initial dose and titrate to desired effect by increasing 2.5 mg/h every 5 minutes to max of 15 mg/h; if blood pressure is not controlled by nicardipine, consider sodium nitroprusside
Systolic 180 to 230 **or** diastolic 105 to 120	• Labetalol 10 mg IV for 1 to 2 minutes • May repeat or double labetalol every 10 to 20 minutes to max dose of 300 mg, or give initial labetalol dose, then start labetalol drip at 2 to 8 mg/min

Transfer to General or Intensive Care

All patients with stroke should be admitted to a stroke unit (if available) for careful monitoring of blood pressure, neurologic status, and treatment of hypertension if indicated (as above). General care for stroke patients includes the following:

- Support the airway, oxygenation and ventilation, and nutritional status.
- Administer IV normal saline at approximately 75 to 100 mL/h to maintain intravascular volume if needed.
- Consider management of hyperglycemia when the blood glucose is above 200 mg/dL.
- Treat fever. Hyperthermia is associated with increased morbidity and mortality. Induced hypothermia has not been shown beneficial in controlled human clinical trials.
- If the patient's neurologic status deteriorates, order a repeat CT scan to determine if cerebral edema or hemorrhage has caused the deterioration.

Appendix A

Skill Station Competency Checklist **Management of Respiratory Arrest**	☑ if done correctly

BLS Primary Survey and Interventions	
Establishes unresponsiveness • Activates EMS and gets AED *or* • Directs 2nd rescuer to activate the emergency response system and get the AED	
• Opens the airway (head tilt–chin lift or, if trauma is suspected, jaw thrust without head extension) • Checks for breathing (look, listen, and feel; at least 5 seconds but not more than 10 seconds)	
If breathing is absent or inadequate, gives 2 breaths (1 second per breath) that cause the chest to rise	
Checks carotid pulse. Notes that pulse is present. Does not initiate chest compressions or attach AED. Performs rescue breaths at the correct rate of 1 breath every 5 to 6 seconds (10 to 12 breaths/min)	
ACLS Secondary Survey Case Skills	
Inserts oropharyngeal and nasopharyngeal airway (student should demonstrate both)	
Performs correct bag-mask ventilation	
Administers oxygen	
Reassesses pulse about every 2 minutes	
CRITICAL ACTIONS	
Performs Primary ABCDs	
Properly inserts OPA or NPA	
Can ventilate with bag-mask	
Gives proper ventilation—rate and volume	
Rechecks pulse and other sign of circulation. Does not initiate chest compressions.	

CPR/AED Testing Checklist

VF Treated With CPR and Automated External Defibrillation (1 Rescuer)

Skill Step	CRITICAL PERFORMANCE STEPS	Adult/Child CPR With AED ☑ if done correctly
1	Checks unresponsiveness	
2	Tells someone to activate EMS and get an AED	
3	Opens airway using head tilt–chin lift	
4	Checks breathing *Minimum 5 seconds; maximum 10 seconds*	
5	Gives 2 breaths (1 second each)	
6	Checks carotid pulse *Minimum 5 seconds; maximum 10 seconds*	
7	Locates CPR hand position	
8	Delivers first cycle of compressions at correct rate *Acceptable <23 sec for 30 compressions*	
9	Gives 2 breaths (1 second each)	
AED arrives		
AED 1	Turns AED on	
AED 2	Selects proper AED pads and places pads correctly	
AED 3	Clears patient to analyze *(must be visible and verbal check)*	
AED 4	Clears patient to shock/presses shock button *(must be visible and verbal check)* *Maximum time from AED arrival <90 sec*	
Student continues CPR		
10	Delivers second cycle of compressions at correct hand position *Acceptable >23 of 30*	
11	Gives 2 breaths (1 second each) with visible chest rise	
The next step is done only with a manikin with a feedback device, such as a clicker or light. If not, STOP THE TEST.		
12	Delivers third cycle of compressions of adequate depth with full chest recoil *Acceptable >23 compressions*	

TEST RESULTS	Indicate Pass or Needs Remediation:	P	NR
Instructor signature affirms that skills tests were done according to AHA guidelines. *Save this sheet with course record.*	Instructor Signature: _____ Print Inst. Name: _____ Date: _____		

Learning Station Competency Checklist

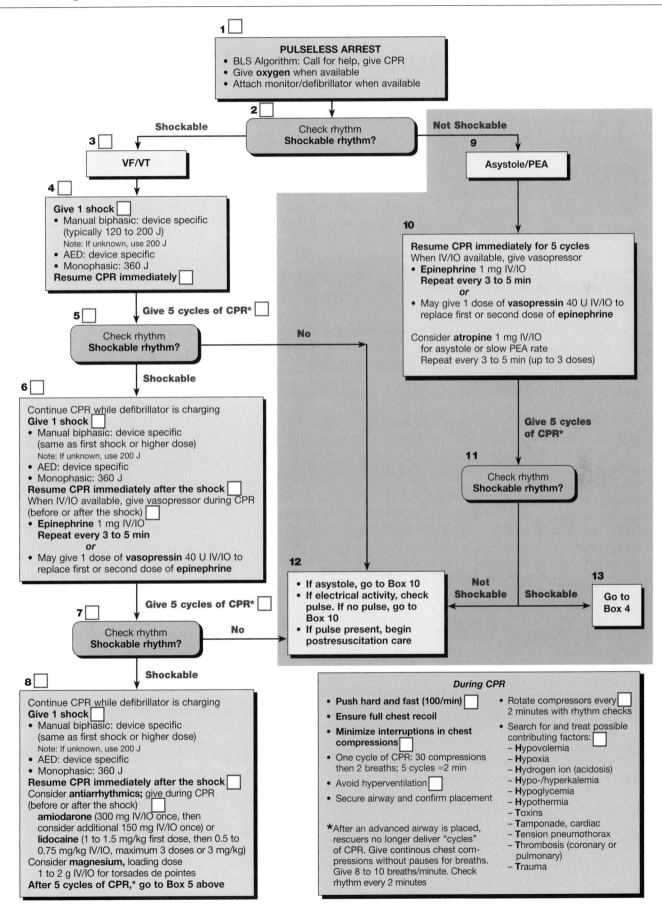

1 ☐
PULSELESS ARREST
- BLS Algorithm: Call for help, give CPR
- Give **oxygen** when available
- Attach monitor/defibrillator when available

2 ☐
Check rhythm
Shockable rhythm?

Shockable →

Not Shockable

3 ☐
VF/VT

9
Asystole/PEA

4 ☐
Give 1 shock ☐
- Manual biphasic: device specific (typically 120 to 200 J)
  Note: If unknown, use 200 J
- AED: device specific
- Monophasic: 360 J
Resume CPR immediately ☐

10
Resume CPR immediately for 5 cycles
When IV/IO available, give vasopressor
- **Epinephrine** 1 mg IV/IO
  Repeat every 3 to 5 min
  or
- May give 1 dose of **vasopressin** 40 U IV/IO to replace first or second dose of **epinephrine**

Consider **atropine** 1 mg IV/IO
  for asystole or slow PEA rate
  Repeat every 3 to 5 min (up to 3 doses)

Give 5 cycles of CPR* ☐

5 ☐
Check rhythm
Shockable rhythm?

No →

Shockable

6 ☐
Continue CPR while defibrillator is charging
Give 1 shock ☐
- Manual biphasic: device specific (same as first shock or higher dose)
  Note: If unknown, use 200 J
- AED: device specific
- Monophasic: 360 J
Resume CPR immediately after the shock ☐
When IV/IO available, give vasopressor during CPR (before or after the shock)
- **Epinephrine** 1 mg IV/IO
  Repeat every 3 to 5 min
  or
- May give 1 dose of **vasopressin** 40 U IV/IO to replace first or second dose of **epinephrine**

Give 5 cycles of CPR* ☐

Give 5 cycles of CPR*

11
Check rhythm
Shockable rhythm?

7 ☐
Check rhythm
Shockable rhythm?

No →

Shockable

12
- If asystole, go to Box 10
- If electrical activity, check pulse. If no pulse, go to Box 10
- If pulse present, begin postresuscitation care

Not Shockable ←

Shockable →

13
Go to Box 4

8 ☐
Continue CPR while defibrillator is charging
Give 1 shock ☐
- Manual biphasic: device specific (same as first shock or higher dose)
  Note: If unknown, use 200 J
- AED: device specific
- Monophasic: 360 J
Resume CPR immediately after the shock ☐
Consider **antiarrhythmics;** give during CPR (before or after the shock) ☐
  amiodarone (300 mg IV/IO once, then consider additional 150 mg IV/IO once) or
  lidocaine (1 to 1.5 mg/kg first dose, then 0.5 to 0.75 mg/kg IV/IO, maximum 3 doses or 3 mg/kg)
Consider **magnesium,** loading dose
  1 to 2 g IV/IO for torsades de pointes
After 5 cycles of CPR,* go to Box 5 above

During CPR
- **Push hard and fast (100/min)** ☐
- **Ensure full chest recoil**
- **Minimize interruptions in chest compressions** ☐
- One cycle of CPR: 30 compressions then 2 breaths; 5 cycles ≈2 min
- Avoid hyperventilation ☐
- Secure airway and confirm placement

- Rotate compressors every ☐ 2 minutes with rhythm checks
- Search for and treat possible contributing factors: ☐
  – **H**ypovolemia
  – **H**ypoxia
  – **H**ydrogen ion (acidosis)
  – **H**ypo-/hyperkalemia
  – **H**ypoglycemia
  – **H**ypothermia
  – **T**oxins
  – **T**amponade, cardiac
  – **T**ension pneumothorax
  – **T**hrombosis (coronary or pulmonary)
  – **T**rauma

*After an advanced airway is placed, rescuers no longer deliver "cycles" of CPR. Give continous chest compressions without pauses for breaths. Give 8 to 10 breaths/minute. Check rhythm every 2 minutes

Learning Station Competency Checklist

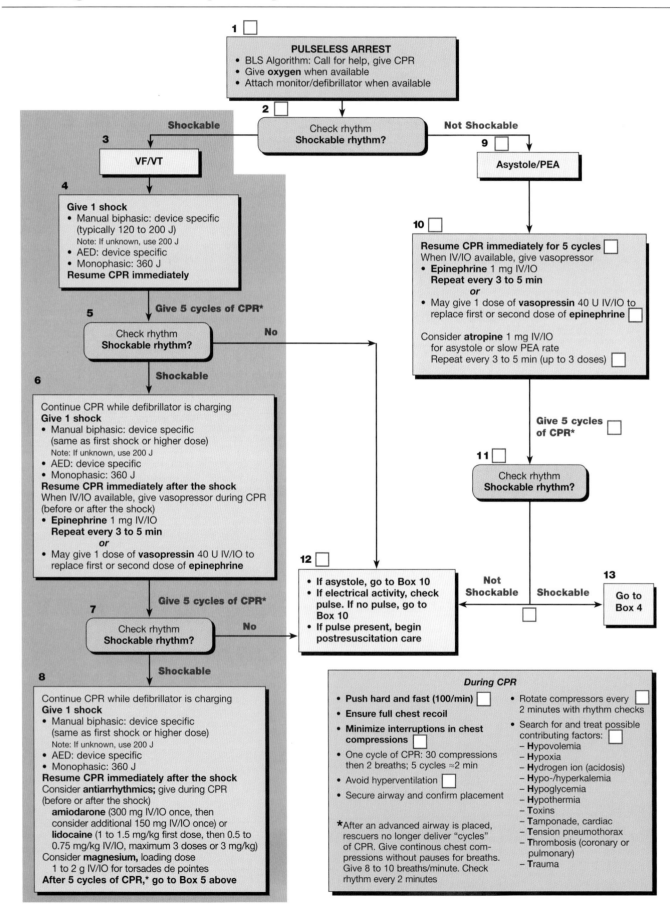

1 ☐

PULSELESS ARREST
- BLS Algorithm: Call for help, give CPR
- Give **oxygen** when available
- Attach monitor/defibrillator when available

2 ☐

Check rhythm
Shockable rhythm?

Shockable →

← Not Shockable

3

VF/VT

9 ☐

Asystole/PEA

4

Give 1 shock
- Manual biphasic: device specific (typically 120 to 200 J)
  Note: If unknown, use 200 J
- AED: device specific
- Monophasic: 360 J
Resume CPR immediately

Give 5 cycles of CPR*

5

Check rhythm
Shockable rhythm?

No →

↓ Shockable

6

Continue CPR while defibrillator is charging
Give 1 shock
- Manual biphasic: device specific (same as first shock or higher dose)
  Note: If unknown, use 200 J
- AED: device specific
- Monophasic: 360 J
Resume CPR immediately after the shock
When IV/IO available, give vasopressor during CPR (before or after the shock)
- **Epinephrine** 1 mg IV/IO
  Repeat every 3 to 5 min
      or
- May give 1 dose of **vasopressin** 40 U IV/IO to replace first or second dose of **epinephrine**

Give 5 cycles of CPR*

7

Check rhythm
Shockable rhythm?

No →

↓ Shockable

8

Continue CPR while defibrillator is charging
Give 1 shock
- Manual biphasic: device specific (same as first shock or higher dose)
  Note: If unknown, use 200 J
- AED: device specific
- Monophasic: 360 J
Resume CPR immediately after the shock
Consider **antiarrhythmics;** give during CPR (before or after the shock)
   amiodarone (300 mg IV/IO once, then consider additional 150 mg IV/IO once) or
   lidocaine (1 to 1.5 mg/kg first dose, then 0.5 to 0.75 mg/kg IV/IO, maximum 3 doses or 3 mg/kg)
Consider **magnesium,** loading dose 1 to 2 g IV/IO for torsades de pointes
After 5 cycles of CPR,* go to Box 5 above

10 ☐

Resume CPR immediately for 5 cycles ☐
When IV/IO available, give vasopressor
- **Epinephrine** 1 mg IV/IO
  Repeat every 3 to 5 min
      or
- May give 1 dose of **vasopressin** 40 U IV/IO to replace first or second dose of **epinephrine ☐**

Consider **atropine** 1 mg IV/IO
for asystole or slow PEA rate
Repeat every 3 to 5 min (up to 3 doses) ☐

Give 5 cycles ☐ of CPR*

11 ☐

Check rhythm
Shockable rhythm?

12 ☐
- If asystole, go to Box 10
- If electrical activity, check pulse. If no pulse, go to Box 10
- If pulse present, begin postresuscitation care

Not Shockable ←   Shockable →

13

Go to Box 4

During CPR

- **Push hard and fast (100/min) ☐**
- **Ensure full chest recoil**
- **Minimize interruptions in chest compressions ☐**
- One cycle of CPR: 30 compressions then 2 breaths; 5 cycles ≈2 min
- Avoid hyperventilation ☐
- Secure airway and confirm placement

*After an advanced airway is placed, rescuers no longer deliver "cycles" of CPR. Give continuous chest compressions without pauses for breaths. Give 8 to 10 breaths/minute. Check rhythm every 2 minutes

- Rotate compressors every ☐ 2 minutes with rhythm checks
- Search for and treat possible contributing factors: ☐
  – **H**ypovolemia
  – **H**ypoxia
  – **H**ydrogen ion (acidosis)
  – **H**ypo-/hyperkalemia
  – **H**ypoglycemia
  – **H**ypothermia
  – **T**oxins
  – **T**amponade, cardiac
  – **T**ension pneumothorax
  – **T**hrombosis (coronary or pulmonary)
  – **T**rauma

Learning Station Competency Checklist

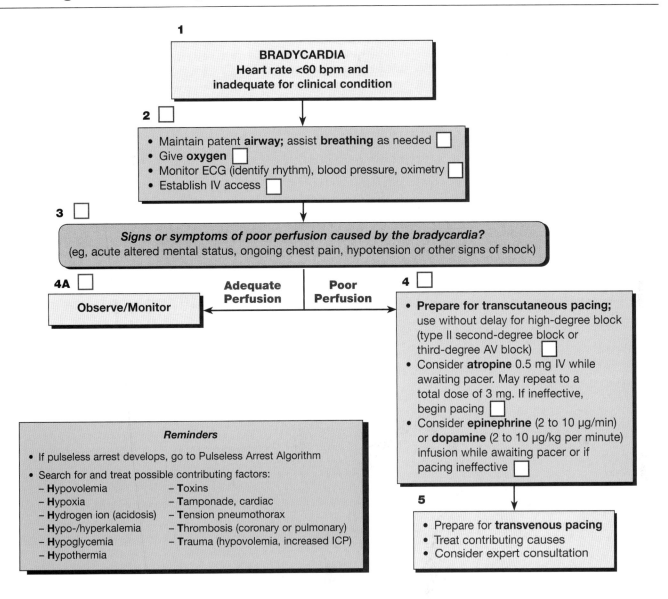

1

BRADYCARDIA
Heart rate <60 bpm and
inadequate for clinical condition

2 ☐

- Maintain patent **airway;** assist **breathing** as needed ☐
- Give **oxygen** ☐
- Monitor ECG (identify rhythm), blood pressure, oximetry ☐
- Establish IV access ☐

3 ☐

Signs or symptoms of poor perfusion caused by the bradycardia?
(eg, acute altered mental status, ongoing chest pain, hypotension or other signs of shock)

4A ☐   **Adequate Perfusion**   **Poor Perfusion**   **4** ☐

Observe/Monitor

- **Prepare for transcutaneous pacing;** use without delay for high-degree block (type II second-degree block or third-degree AV block) ☐
- Consider **atropine** 0.5 mg IV while awaiting pacer. May repeat to a total dose of 3 mg. If ineffective, begin pacing ☐
- Consider **epinephrine** (2 to 10 µg/min) or **dopamine** (2 to 10 µg/kg per minute) infusion while awaiting pacer or if pacing ineffective ☐

Reminders

- If pulseless arrest develops, go to Pulseless Arrest Algorithm
- Search for and treat possible contributing factors:
  - **H**ypovolemia
  - **H**ypoxia
  - **H**ydrogen ion (acidosis)
  - **H**ypo-/hyperkalemia
  - **H**ypoglycemia
  - **H**ypothermia
  - **T**oxins
  - **T**amponade, cardiac
  - **T**ension pneumothorax
  - **T**hrombosis (coronary or pulmonary)
  - **T**rauma (hypovolemia, increased ICP)

5

- Prepare for **transvenous pacing**
- Treat contributing causes
- Consider expert consultation

Learning Station Competency Checklist

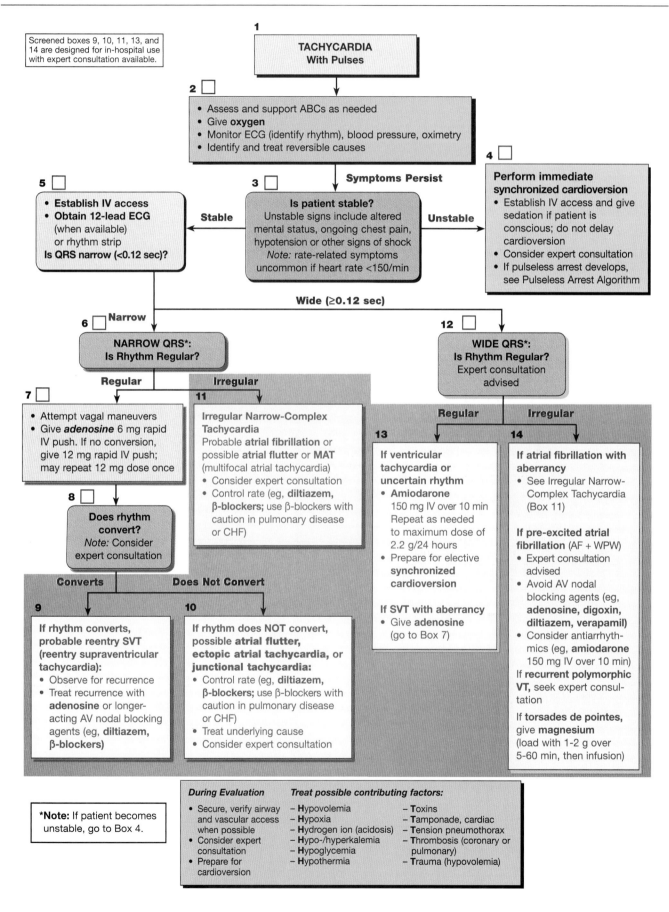

Screened boxes 9, 10, 11, 13, and 14 are designed for in-hospital use with expert consultation available.

1
**TACHYCARDIA
With Pulses**

2
- Assess and support ABCs as needed
- Give **oxygen**
- Monitor ECG (identify rhythm), blood pressure, oximetry
- Identify and treat reversible causes

Symptoms Persist

4
Perform immediate synchronized cardioversion
- Establish IV access and give sedation if patient is conscious; do not delay cardioversion
- Consider expert consultation
- If pulseless arrest develops, see Pulseless Arrest Algorithm

5
- **Establish IV access**
- **Obtain 12-lead ECG**
  (when available)
  or rhythm strip
Is QRS narrow (<0.12 sec)?

Stable

3
Is patient stable?
Unstable signs include altered mental status, ongoing chest pain, hypotension or other signs of shock
Note: rate-related symptoms uncommon if heart rate <150/min

Unstable

Wide (≥0.12 sec)

Narrow

6
**NARROW QRS*:
Is Rhythm Regular?**

12
**WIDE QRS*:
Is Rhythm Regular?**
Expert consultation advised

Regular

Irregular

7
- Attempt vagal maneuvers
- Give *adenosine* 6 mg rapid IV push. If no conversion, give 12 mg rapid IV push; may repeat 12 mg dose once

11
Irregular Narrow-Complex Tachycardia
Probable **atrial fibrillation** or possible **atrial flutter** or **MAT** (multifocal atrial tachycardia)
- Consider expert consultation
- Control rate (eg, **diltiazem, β-blockers;** use β-blockers with caution in pulmonary disease or CHF)

Regular

Irregular

13
If ventricular tachycardia or uncertain rhythm
- **Amiodarone**
  150 mg IV over 10 min Repeat as needed to maximum dose of 2.2 g/24 hours
- Prepare for elective **synchronized cardioversion**

If SVT with aberrancy
- Give **adenosine** (go to Box 7)

14
If atrial fibrillation with aberrancy
- See Irregular Narrow-Complex Tachycardia (Box 11)

If pre-excited atrial fibrillation (AF + WPW)
- Expert consultation advised
- Avoid AV nodal blocking agents (eg, **adenosine, digoxin, diltiazem, verapamil**)
- Consider antiarrhythmics (eg, **amiodarone** 150 mg IV over 10 min)
If **recurrent polymorphic VT,** seek expert consultation

If **torsades de pointes,** give **magnesium** (load with 1-2 g over 5-60 min, then infusion)

8
Does rhythm convert?
Note: Consider expert consultation

Converts

Does Not Convert

9
If rhythm converts, probable reentry SVT (reentry supraventricular tachycardia):
- Observe for recurrence
- Treat recurrence with **adenosine** or longer-acting AV nodal blocking agents (eg, **diltiazem, β-blockers**)

10
If rhythm does NOT convert, possible atrial flutter, ectopic atrial tachycardia, or **junctional tachycardia:**
- Control rate (eg, **diltiazem, β-blockers;** use β-blockers with caution in pulmonary disease or CHF)
- Treat underlying cause
- Consider expert consultation

*Note: If patient becomes unstable, go to Box 4.

During Evaluation
- Secure, verify airway and vascular access when possible
- Consider expert consultation
- Prepare for cardioversion

Treat possible contributing factors:
- **H**ypovolemia
- **H**ypoxia
- **H**ydrogen ion (acidosis)
- **H**ypo-/hyperkalemia
- **H**ypoglycemia
- **H**ypothermia

- **T**oxins
- **T**amponade, cardiac
- **T**ension pneumothorax
- **T**hrombosis (coronary or pulmonary)
- **T**rauma (hypovolemia)

Megacode Testing Checklist 1/2
Bradycardia→VF/Pulseless VT→Asystole

Critical Performance Steps	☑ if done correctly
Team Leader	
Ensures high-quality CPR at all times	
Assigns team member roles	
Bradycardia Management	
Starts oxygen, places monitor, starts IV	
Places monitor leads in proper position	
Recognizes symptomatic bradycardia	
Administers appropriate drug(s) and doses	
Verbalizes the need for TCP	
VF/Pulseless VT Management	
Recognizes VF	
Clears before ANALYZE and SHOCK	
Immediately resumes CPR after shocks	
Appropriate airway management	
Appropriate cycles Drug—Rhythm Check/Shock—CPR	
Administers appropriate drug(s) and doses	
Asystole Management	
Recognizes asystole	
Verbalizes potential reversible causes of Asystole/PEA (H's and T's)	
Administers appropriate drug(s) and doses	
Immediately resumes CPR after rhythm checks	
	STOP THE TEST

TEST RESULTS	Indicate Pass or Needs Remediation:	P	NR
Instructor signature affirms that skills tests were done according to AHA guidelines. *Save this sheet with course record.*	Instructor Signature: _____ Print Inst. Name: _____ Date: _____		

Megacode Testing Checklist 3
Tachycardia→VF/Pulseless VT→PEA

Critical Performance Steps	☑ if done correctly
Team Leader	
Ensures high-quality CPR at all times	
Assigns team member roles	
Tachycardia Management	
Starts oxygen, places monitor, starts IV	
Places monitor leads in proper position	
Recognizes unstable tachycardia	
Recognizes symptoms due to tachycardia	
Performs immediate synchronized cardioversion	
VF/Pulseless VT Management	
Recognizes VF	
Clears before ANALYZE and SHOCK	
Immediately resumes CPR after shocks	
Appropriate airway management	
Appropriate cycles Drug—Rhythm Check/Shock—CPR	
Administers appropriate drug(s) and doses	
PEA Management	
Recognizes PEA	
Verbalizes potential reversible causes of PEA/asystole (H's and T's)	
Administers appropriate drug(s) and doses	
Immediately resumes CPR after rhythm and pulse checks	
	STOP THE TEST

TEST RESULTS	Indicate Pass or Needs Remediation:	P	NR
Instructor signature affirms that skills tests were done according to AHA guidelines. *Save this sheet with course record.*	Instructor Signature: _____ Print Inst. Name: _____ Date: _____		

Megacode Testing Checklist 4
Tachycardia→VF/Pulseless VT→PEA

Critical Performance Steps	☑ if done correctly
Team Leader	
Ensures high-quality CPR at all times	
Assigns team member roles	
Tachycardia Management	
Starts oxygen, places monitor, starts IV	
Places monitor leads in proper position	
Recognizes tachycardia (specific diagnosis)	
Recognizes no symptoms due to tachycardia	
Attempts vagal maneuvers	
Gives appropriate initial drug therapy	
VF/Pulseless VT Management	
Recognizes VF	
Clears before ANALYZE and SHOCK	
Immediately resumes CPR after shocks	
Appropriate airway management	
Appropriate cycles Drug—Rhythm Check/Shock—CPR	
Administers appropriate drug(s) and doses	
PEA Management	
Recognizes PEA	
Verbalizes potential reversible causes of PEA/asystole (H's and T's)	
Administers appropriate drug(s) and doses	
Immediately resumes CPR after rhythm and pulse checks	
	STOP THE TEST

TEST RESULTS	Indicate Pass or Needs Remediation:	P	NR
Instructor signature affirms that skills tests were done according to AHA guidelines. *Save this sheet with course record.*	Instructor Signature: _____ Print Inst. Name: _____ Date: _____		

Appendix B

ACLS Science Overview Worksheet

Use this worksheet to take notes on the science changes that are mentioned in the ACLS Science Overview Video.

Topic	Notes
Basic Life Support/CPR	**1. Effective Chest Compressions** Rate Coronary perfusion pressure Key concepts • *Push hard and fast* • *Allow full chest recoil* • *Minimize interruptions in compressions* • *Avoid hyperventilation* **2. Compression-to-ventilation ratio** Ratio Interruptions **3. Rescue breaths** Delivery Volume Danger of hyperventilation

Topic	Notes
ACLS	**1. Defibrillation** How many shocks? Why? Follow with compressions. Why? When to check for a pulse Organizing drug therapy The ECG When recommendations may be modified **2. Witnessed or unwitnessed cardiac arrest** Call-to-arrival interval Shock dose
CPR Interruptions	**1. Responsibilities of team leader** **2. Weighing the need for an advanced airway** **3. After an advanced airway is in place** **4. Confirming endotracheal tube placement** **5. IV/IO drug administration**
ACLS Pulseless Arrest Algorithm	**1. Treatment sequence** Continuous CPR Number of shocks When to perform rhythm checks Preparing drugs **2. Difference in sequence if in-hospital**

ACLS Course Overview

ACLS Course Design

Scientific evidence has pointed the way toward better ACLS course content. Educational research has pointed the way toward better ACLS course design. AHA's ACLS course is evidence-based.

ACLS Course Overview

The ACLS course is designed to emphasize three major concepts:

- The importance of basic life support CPR to patient survival
- The integration of effective BLS with ACLS interventions
- The importance of effective team interaction and communication during resuscitation

The Importance of CPR

Science shows that effective CPR (proper chest compressions and ventilations) are more important than drugs for cardiac arrest survival. CPR is not performed well by rescuers during out-of-hospital and in-hospital arrests. CPR skills retention studies have shown a consistent pattern of significant erosion of CPR skills in days, weeks, and months after a CPR course.

Continuous, effective CPR is the foundation for ACLS and should never be compromised. All ACLS students are expected to perform CPR effectively and competently throughout the course. ACLS emphasizes core BLS principles:

- Push hard and fast (100 per minute)
- Minimize interruptions in compressions
- Allow full chest recoil between compressions
- Avoid hyperventilation

ACLS Skills

Saving a cardiac arrest patient requires cognitive and psychomotor skills.

Cognitive	Psychomotor
Rhythms	Compressions
Drugs	Ventilations
Algorithms	Basic and advanced airway management

ACLS and BLS Skills Integration

ACLS interventions are add-ons to the core skills of BLS and must be carefully integrated into ongoing BLS efforts. If you do not perform good BLS, there is a strong probability that your ACLS efforts may fail.

Pulseless Arrest Diagram

The following is the pulseless arrest diagram:

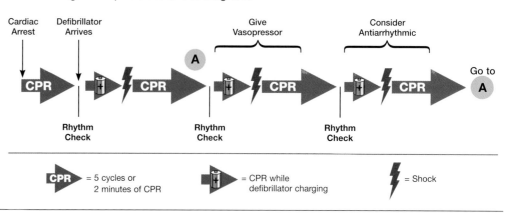

Team Resuscitation Approach

A team approach increases resuscitation success. A team leader is responsible for ensuring that things get done in the right way at the right time. Team members are proficient in skills (within their scope of practice). Effective teamwork and communication increases resuscitation success.

The ACLS course emphasizes the Team Approach. You will learn and practice being a team leader in simulated cases. You will perform all team member roles in simulated cases.

What You Will Do in This Course

You will do the following in this course:

- Learn and practice specific skills in Learning Stations
- Integrate these skills in simulated cases
- Practice and be proficient in managing a "megacode" as a team leader

ACLS Course Completion Requirements

To successfully complete this ACLS course, students must

- Actively participate in, practice, and complete the Learning Stations in the course:
  - Management of Respiratory Arrest
  - Pulseless Arrest VF/VT
  - ACS
  - Bradycardia/Asystole/PEA
  - Stable and Unstable Tachycardia
  - Stroke
- Pass a skills test in 1-rescuer CPR and use of an AED
- Pass a written exam with a minimum score of 84%
- Pass a Megacode Station Test (VF/Pulseless VT and 2 other rhythms)

Index